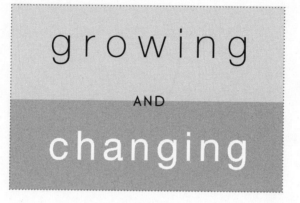

Revised and Updated

growing

AND

changing

Revised and Updated

KATHY MCCOY, Ph.D., and
CHARLES WIBBELSMAN, M.D.

A PERIGEE BOOK

A Perigee Book
Published by The Berkley Publishing Group
A division of Penguin Group (USA) Inc.
375 Hudson Street
New York, New York 10014

First Perigee edition:
Revised and updated edition: August 2003

Library of Congress Cataloging-in-Publication Data

McCoy, Kathy, 1945-
    Growing and changing / Kathy McCoy and Charles Wibbelsman.—Rev. and updated ed.
    p. cm.
    "A Perigee book."
    Includes index.
    Summary: Addresses questions pre-teens have about puberty in such areas as body
changes, changes in feelings, hygiene, health problems, and talking to doctors and parents.
    ISBN 0-399-52898-9
    1. Sex instruction for children. 2. Puberty—Juvenile literature. 3. Children—Health
and hygiene—Juvenile literature. [1. Puberty. 2. Grooming. 3. Health.] I. Wibbelsman,
Charles. II. Title.

HQ53.M44 2003
649'.65—dc21

2003042918

Printed in the United States of America

10 9 8 7 6 5 4 3 2 1

Table of Contents

What Is Puberty?

What does puberty mean? My brother, who is 16, says it means getting pimples and growing taller and more muscular. My mom says it means you start thinking you know everything and your parents know nothing. My sister (she's 14) says it means you could have children of your own. My dad doesn't say much of anything except that I'll know what it means when I'm old enough. I'm 10 years old and wonder a lot about what's going to happen to me, even though right now I don't have any signs of growing up that I can see. ✻ JASON R.

Will someone tell me what's going on? My doctor keeps weighing and measuring me every time I see him. He says my body will start changing a lot pretty soon. What's supposed to happen when you're my age (almost 11)? ✻ GERALD B.

I'm 11, and my two best friends look much more mature than I do. They wear bras. (My mother won't let me get one because she says I don't need it yet. I'm totally FLAT! But I wish I had a bra anyway.) What I want to know is this: How can I tell when I'm going to go through the changes my friends are experiencing already? So far, I don't have any noticeable signs of maturity. Am I normal anyway? ✻ MICHELLE K.

Puberty is the time of your life when you grow from childhood to young adulthood. Puberty is a special time. It can also be a confusing time. Why? Because so much in your life is changing.

Your body is growing taller and changing its shape. If you're a boy, you will be getting broader shoulders and more noticeable muscles. If you're a girl, your hips are getting broader and your whole body is becoming softer and rounded. You may have, or will soon begin to develop, some physical traits of adulthood such as hair under your arms, in the area between your legs and on your legs. During puberty, girls develop breasts and begin to menstruate. Boys notice their penis and testicles growing. These are all important changes.

As we will see in the chapters to come, these physical changes don't happen overnight or in quite the same way for everyone. It usually takes at least several years for all of the changes to occur. Some boys and girls go through puberty at a fairly young age, starting to show noticeable signs of growing up as early as 8 or 9. This is normal for them. Those who start the changes of puberty at a later age are also normal.

Whenever puberty starts for you, it means that you're gradually getting ready to live the life of an adult. Your body is getting the stature and strength to do adult things—from driving a car to doing hard physical work. Your body changes are also preparing you to have children of your own someday. For now, the signs of puberty mean that you're well on your way to young adulthood!

There are other important changes that happen at this time that aren't physical. Some of your feelings and interests may be changing, too. Your friends are probably becoming more and more important to you. You may be starting to notice the opposite sex with new interest. You may find yourself becoming more and more independent. You may want to have more say these days in choosing your clothes or friends or activities. You're learning, more and more, how to take care of yourself and how to make decisions on your own. That's all part of growing up.

But growing up is a process that starts long before the dramatic changes we call puberty. Just as you learn skills throughout your childhood that will someday help you to live on your own, so your body starts preparing for puberty long before you have any outward signs of growing up.

How does this process of growing up begin?

It all starts in your brain with changes you can't see or feel. These invisible changes usually take place several years before you notice your body actually growing and changing. What happens?

The pituitary gland (see Fig. 1-1), which is the master control gland of the body, begins to send a special hormone into your bloodstream. This special signal alerts some other glands—your ovaries if you are a girl, your testicles if you are a boy—to start producing the hormones that will make all your physical changes of puberty possible. In girls, this hormone is estrogen. Boys produce testosterone. As you get closer and closer to the time when puberty will begin, the amount of these hormones in your body will increase.

It is estrogen or testosterone that will make your breasts or penis and testicles grow.

These hormones will also cause you to grow taller and to develop the body shape of a young man or woman.

These hormones will cause pubic, leg and underarm hair to grow in both sexes and facial hair to grow in boys.

These hormones will also make perspiration glands and the oil glands of your skin become more active, meaning that you will perspire more under your arms and notice your skin becoming oily.

These hormones will cause your voice to change so you begin to sound more like an adult. Both boys and girls experience a voice change, but it's much more noticeable in boys.

So even if you haven't noticed any outward signs of puberty, wonderful things may already be happening inside as your body begins to

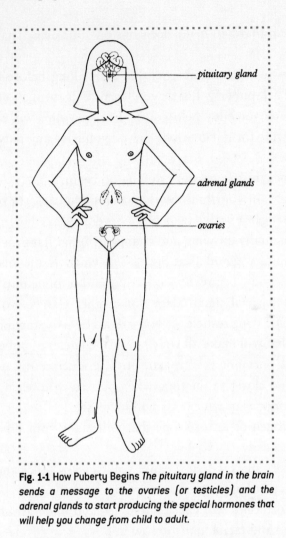

Fig. 1-1 How Puberty Begins *The pituitary gland in the brain sends a message to the ovaries (or testicles) and the adrenal glands to start producing the special hormones that will help you change from child to adult.*

produce the hormones that make it possible for you to grow into an adult man or woman.

Some people think puberty is just a big problem, that it means pimples and feeling upset and embarrassed a lot of the time. Some young people do get acne. And, if you're like most people, there will be times when you are embarrassed or confused by all the changes taking place in your life. But puberty is also a sign to you and everyone around you that you're *really* growing up. And that can lead to new privileges, new strengths and skills, new friends, new experiences and, gradually, more personal freedom.

At those times when some of the changes in your body, your feelings and your life seem very strange and confusing, it's important to remember that puberty is a natural part of life. Everyone goes through it. Everyone worries about being normal. Everyone has questions.

That's why we're writing this book just for you. We want you to know that you're not alone. We want you to understand what's happening inside and outside your body during these important years of change. We want to help you learn what's normal for you and what to expect so you can look forward to and feel comfortable with each change. When you know more, you'll feel even *better* about growing up!

When Will My Body Start Changing?

I still look like a kid. But all my friends look like teenagers already. It's embarrassing! Is it normal to be slower to grow up than my friends? Is something wrong with me? I'm 12 already! When will my body start changing? ✳ SARAH G.

What makes one person show signs of growing up before another? I'm taller and four months older than my best friend, but she got her period first! She's still 11, but I just turned 12. So what's going on? ✳ EMILY A.

Each person has his or her own normal biological time clock for starting puberty. For some girls, the starting time for these physical changes is as early as 7 or 8. Sometimes this is a result of your ethnicity. For example, studies show that nearly half of all African American girls begin the changes of puberty—changes like the beginning of breast development or the first signs of pubic hair growth—by the age of 8 (compared with 15 percent of white girls.) No one knows for sure why African American girls often appear to grow up faster than girls in other ethnic groups. Some researchers think that exposure to chemicals that mimic or contain the female hormone estrogen may be a cause. Such chemicals are sometimes found in milk and meat and also in some hair products made specifically for African Americans. Some researchers feel that stress, including the stress of being a racial or ethnic minority in a still-racist society, could be serious enough to make some girls mature more quickly than others.

Some medical experts feel that the easy availability of nutritious food (as well as junk food) is making young people look older sooner. If you could travel back in time 100 years ago or so, you'd notice that 16- and 17-year-olds looked pretty much like some of your friends do today. At the turn of the century, it wasn't at all unusual for a girl not to get her period until she was 17. Today, the average age is about 12. Along these same nutritional lines, medical experts have noted that very overweight or obese girls tend to start puberty sooner than their more slender friends.

Of course, in many cases, the timing of puberty is hereditary, and this can be true for both boys and girls. You may start noticing the first signs of physical change at about the same age your mom or dad did. (So if that is the kind of thing you can imagine discussing with your parents, you could learn a lot about what to expect with your own physical changes!)

For example, if your dad didn't start to show any of the changes of growing up until he was pretty well into his teens, you may follow the same timetable. If he started puberty at an earlier-than-average age, you may, too. Resembling a parent in this way is as normal as inheriting his or her eye color or type of hair.

So chances are that your progress through puberty, as unique and individual as your personal time clock is, is entirely normal.

But even though you're normal inside, you may feel very different as you look around at your friends. Maybe your rate of growth is faster or slower than theirs. Maybe you aren't experiencing one or two of the changes you see in your friends. Maybe you're beginning to wonder if you're normal.

If you're wondering "Am I normal?" you're not alone! That's the question young people most often ask themselves, their parents and their doctors during these growing years. It's important to remember that most people are both different *and* normal. Your normal rate of physical development is as unique as your personality. It's not quite like anyone else's.

If you're worried about being normal, it might help to talk with your parents or your doctor. Your parents might give you some helpful information about their own growing up that could explain why you are maturing earlier or later than your friends. Your doctor or school nurse can give you lots of facts about the very normal, very individual changes of puberty.

Puberty Talk: What Does It Mean?

I'm 12 and scared. And I'm confused, too. I went to my doctor for a checkup yesterday, and he told my mother some stuff I didn't under-stand. He said my testickals (?) are growing and that pretty soon I may get pubic and anksillery (spelling?) hair! Are these things normal, or are they problems? What do these words mean? I was too embar-rassed to ask either my doctor or my mom directly. ✻ JIM L.

When grown-ups—whether they're doctors, parents or teachers—talk about puberty, they often use words that may sound very strange to you at first. In order to understand what they're saying, you need to know what all these new words mean. There may be some you know already, but we're including a list of the words you'll see in the rest of this chapter as we discuss the stages of development or words you're likely to hear when those close to you talk about the physical changes of puberty.

■ **areola** (a-ree-**oh**-la): The circle of darker skin surrounding the nipple in both male and female breasts.

■ **axillary** (ak-sil-ler-ee) **hair:** Hair under the arms.

■ **breast buds:** The beginning of breast development in girls. This happens when tissue just under the nipple elevates slightly.

■ **ejaculation** (e-**jack**-you-lay-shun): The release of seminal fluid and sperm from the penis. This usually happens for the first time when a boy is well into puberty.

■ **erection** (e-**reck**-shun): The stiffening of the penis when blood fills the spongy tissues inside it. This often occurs because of sexual excitement, but, especially during puberty, it can happen for no special reason at all.

■ **estrogen** (es-tro-jen): The female sex hormone that makes the physical changes of puberty possible for a girl.

■ **genitals** (**jen**-it-als): The external sex organs that clearly show the difference between boys and girls.

■ **menarche** (men-ark-ee): The beginning of menstruation in a young girl.

■ **menstruation** (men-stroo-**ay**-shun): The normal, healthy process by which the lining of the uterus is shed each month. Menstruation starts during puberty and usually lasts until a woman is in her late forties or early fifties. Women often call menstruation their "menstrual period" or just "period" for short.

■ **nocturnal emission:** Ejaculation during sleep. This is also called a "wet dream." It most often happens to adolescent boys who are not yet sexually active in any way and is the body's way of making room for newer sperm cells.

■ **ovaries** (**oh**-vah-rees): These are two small organs inside a female's abdomen. They are on either side of her uterus. The ovaries are very tiny, but important because they produce the egg cells that will be the woman's contribution in creating any future babies.

■ **ovulation** (ah-view-**lay**-shun): The monthly process by which a ripe egg cell is released from the ovary and travels through the fallopian tube to the uterus.

■ **penis** (**pee**-niss): The male sex organ. The penis is made up of spongy tissues with lots of blood vessels. When these blood vessels fill up and expand, the penis gets stiff—a process called erection.

■ **prostate** (**pross**-state) **gland:** This gland, located by the bottom of a man's bladder, makes much of the seminal fluid that carries sperm through the penis and out of the man's body.

■ **puberty** (**pyou**-ber-tee): The period of time during which the body develops from child to young adult.

■ **pubic** (**pyou**-bic) **hair:** Hair that grows around the genitals in physically mature or maturing males and females.

■ **scrotum** (**skroh**-tum): The sac of skin, hanging just under a male's penis, that holds the testicles.

■ **semen** (**see**-men): A thick, white substance made up of sperm and seminal fluid. This is what comes out of a male's penis when he ejaculates.

■ **seminal** (**sem**-in-ul) **fluid:** The milky white fluid that mixes with sperm just before a male ejaculates.

■ **sperm** (**spurm**): These tiny cells, produced in the testicles, are a man's contribution when making a baby. A woman's egg cell and a man's sperm combine to create a new life. A boy is usually well along in his physical development before he starts to produce sperm cells and to ejaculate them out of his penis.

■ **testicles** (teh-stih-culs) or **testes** (test-ees): The two small egg-shaped organs inside the scrotum. As a boy becomes mature, sperm cells are made in the testicles.

■ **testosterone** (tes-**tah**-stuh-ron): The male sex hormone that makes the physical changes of puberty possible for a boy.

■ **uterus** (**you**-ter-us): This is the organ in the female's lower abdomen where babies can grow and develop. Also, the small amount of blood and tissue that leave her body during menstruation comes from the uterus.

■ **vagina** (vah-ji-nah): The tubelike passageway from a female uterus to the outside of her body. It is also sometimes called the vaginal canal.

■ **vulva** (**vul**-vah): This is a sort of collective name for a female's external genital organs (the ones that you can see).

Now that you know what these words mean, learning about all the normal stages and changes of growing up will be much easier!

Growing Through The Stages

I have a question that probably sounds dumb, but here goes: How do you know when you're in puberty for sure? When is it over, and how do you know that? How long does it last? I don't have any older brothers or sisters, and when I ask my parents how long it lasts, they say "Long enough!" or "Too long!" What's the real answer?? ✽ CODY K.

The process of puberty doesn't happen overnight. It involves five growth stages that may go on for a number of years. The process that starts pretty much unseen when female or male hormones start circulating in your system may not finish until you're about 18 or 19. Yes, it's true! Even those 15- or 16-year-olds who look so totally grown-up are still experiencing puberty but are simply at a more advanced stage than you may be. Each stage of puberty is a temporary way of being on your way to becoming a more grown-up *you*. Your body will go through many temporary ways of being before you settle into your new grown-up look (see Figs. 2-1 to 2-8 of both girls and boys growing from being children to being young men and women).

Even though the stages of puberty have some definite milestones, identified by a British doctor named J. M. Tanner, each person's journey through puberty is unique in some ways. For example, some people's first noticeable growth spurt is in their feet! Their feet grow to adult size before they start to grow in height, and for what seems like forever, they're stumbling around with big adult feet stuck at the end of skinny children's legs! Then, with time, their legs and other body parts begin to grow and change until everything looks just right.

Some people go through the changes of puberty very slowly, while others progress at a faster pace. All are normal. But this means that friends may look temporarily quite different from one another. Your physical changes *do* follow a definite basic pattern, even if they seem, at times, to make absolutely no sense.

The charts on pages 15 and 16 will give you an idea of what the changes of each stage of puberty are and the normal age range for experiencing these.

You may have noticed that, within each stage, there are steps of ongoing changes, like pubic hair growth. At first, it may be sparse and

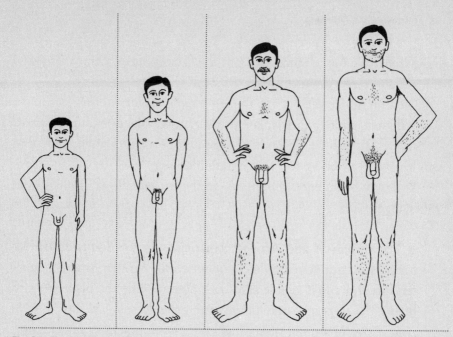

Fig. 2-1, Fig. 2-2, Fig. 2-3, Fig. 2-4 *From Little Boy to Young Man . . . This Is the Way Your Body Will Change and Grow*

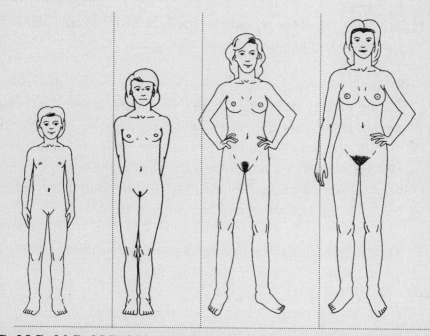

Fig. 2-5, Fig. 2-6, Fig. 2-7, Fig. 2-8 *From Little Girl to Woman . . . This Is the Way Your Body Will Change and Grow*

limited in area, but, as time goes on, it will become darker, coarser and thicker and cover a wider area.

Did you notice the big age range for each stage?

Whether you're an early, late or average bloomer—you're normal.

As we said a little earlier, there are unique aspects of your life that can lead to your being an early or late bloomer.

You may be an early bloomer—on the earlier side of all the physical changes—if:

■ You're female and African American. As we discussed earlier, for reasons not yet completely understood, African American girls tend to show first visible signs of puberty—like the beginnings of breast development and pubic hair growth—as early as 7 or 8! And if you're among these, this early development is entirely normal for you.

■ You are significantly overweight or obese. Studies show that girls who are obese or quite overweight tend to show signs of puberty earlier than their slimmer classmates.

■ You are a person of either gender with a parent or parents who reached puberty at an early age. So if your dad was the tallest in his seventh-grade class and was shaving regularly by the time he reached high school, you may be the same. Or if your mom actually needed a real bra in the fifth grade when all the other girls were begging their moms for "trainer bras" and she started her period before the age of 12, that may be your pattern, too.

You can be a normal late bloomer whose progress through puberty hovers on the late side of each normal age range if:

■ It's in your genes. That is, if one or both parents or other relatives were also late bloomers. This is true for both boys and girls.

What's Going On? Stages of Puberty for Girls

Stages	Ages	Internal	Breasts	Growth	Hair	Menstruation
One	7–11	Ovaries are enlarging and making the hormone estrogen	None	Nothing unusual	None	None
Two	8–14	Estrogen in bloodstream	Breast buds; nipples elevated and tender	Rapid growth; hips broaden; weight gain	First signs: fine, straight and sparse	None
Three	9–15	Vagina is enlarging; chemistry of vaginal secretions changing	Breasts continue to grow; areola enlarges	Height and weight increase	Hair is darker and coarser but is still sparse	First menstrual period may occur at the end of this stage
Four	10–16	Ovaries enlarge; ovulation may begin	Nipple and areola form separate mound	Still growing	Pubic hair looks like an adult's, but covers smaller area; underarm hair appears	First menstrual period now if not at end of stage three; most periods at this stage don't involve ovulation
Five	12–19	Fully mature ovaries; regular ovulation	Full breast development	Full (or near) adult height	Full adult pattern	Regular menstruation with ovulation

What's Going On? Stages of Puberty for Boys

Stages	Ages	Internal	Genitals	Growth	Hair	Maturation
One	9–12	Male hormones active	Nothing obvious; testicles maturing	Some start growth spurt in this stage	No pubic or other body hair	None
Two	9–15	Hormonal changes; muscle and fat to be added to body, changing boy's shape	Testicles, scrotum enlarging; penis is not yet increasing much in size	Rapid growth and changing physique	Pubic hair appears at the base of the penis; will be straight and fine	The areola, the circle of darker skin around each nipple, will increase in size and darken a little
Three	11–16		Penis grows mostly in length; testicles, scrotum growing	Adding more muscle tissue; still growing; shoulders broaden	Pubic hair darker and coarse, spreading along the base of the penis; first traces of hair on upper lip	Voice starts deepening due to growth of larynx
Four	11–17	Sperm production begins; first ejaculation	Penis grows in width; testicles still growing		Underarm and facial hair increases; pubic hair looks more adult	Voice gets deeper and skin becomes more oily
Five	14–18	Full development	Adult in appearance	Near full adult height	Adult pubic hair; full beard	May get chest, body hair later

■ You're below the optimal weight for your height due to strenuous physical activities with stringent weight requirements like ballet, figure skating or gymnastics or if you have an eating disorder
like anorexia nervosa. The fact is, if you're female, you have to
have a certain percentage of body fat in order for the changes of
puberty, like the beginning of menstruation (this is called menarche) to take place. That's why a weight gain and a softening of
your childlike, angular figure usually comes before the most dramatic changes of puberty. (So if you've been stressing about gaining weight, consider that this weight increase could be a normal
part of the changes of puberty.)

When do doctors worry about someone showing signs of puberty
early or late? New guidelines for normal versus "precocious" puberty
would be the presence of breast development or pubic hair growth
before the age of 6 in African American girls and before the age of 7 in
Caucasian girls. For boys, the normal timetable runs a little later—if a
boy shows obvious signs of puberty before the age of 9, he would be
experiencing precocious puberty.

What about late bloomers? When should you start to worry? If
you're a boy and haven't had a sign of testicular growth by the age of
14, you need to check with your doctor. If you're a girl and haven't
had any breast development at all by the age of 13 or begun having
menstrual periods by the age of 15 or 16, you need to have a medical
evaluation. This is also true if you started showing other signs of
puberty within the range of normal but have not menstruated by the
age of 16.

If you feel you're an early or late bloomer, but still fall within the
normal range for the changes of puberty, you may get some reassurance by checking out our age charts.

As you can see from the girls chart, one very normal girl may start
breast development at the age of 8 and have her menarche at age 9 or
10. At the same time, a classmate of hers may not begin breast development until the age of 14 and might not menstruate until she is 16.

Age Range of Changes of Puberty for Boys

CHANGE	8	9	10	11	12	13	14	15	16	17	18	19
Testicle growth	▓	▓	▓	▓	▓	▓	▓					
First pubic hair			▓	▓	▓	▓	▓					
Rapid height increase		▓	▓	▓	▓	▓	▓	▓	▓			
Areola growth					▓	▓	▓	▓				
Penis growth				▓	▓	▓	▓	▓	▓			
Voice deepens					▓	▓	▓	▓	▓	▓		
Armpit, facial hair					▓	▓	▓	▓	▓	▓	▓	
Start sperm production						▓	▓	▓	▓			
Chest, leg and forearm hair growth begin							▓	▓	▓	▓	▓	▓

Looking at the shaded bars for each physical change, you can see that the "normal" range is very wide in most cases.

Take the beginning of breast development, for example. The bar starts at 8 years and reaches to 14. That means that any time within those years is a normal time to start developing breasts.

You can read the boys chart in the same way. Looking at the bars on the chart, you can tell that a boy is likely to get some pubic hair before he gets much penis growth. And all these changes come before his first ejaculation. Look at each of the bars. These mark the normal age span—from early to late bloomer—for each change. Those who have an average rate of growth would be somewhere in the middle of the shaded bar.

Studies by doctors have shown what you may know already if you're an early or late bloomer: It isn't easy to be different! A recent

Age Range of Changes of Puberty for Girls

CHANGE	8	9	10	11	12	13	14	15	16	17	18	19
Hips broaden	▓	▓	▓	▓	▓	▓	▓					
Rapid growth	▓	▓	▓	▓	▓	▓	▓					
First breast development	▓	▓	▓	▓	▓	▓	▓					
First pubic hair		▓	▓	▓	▓	▓	▓	▓				
First menstruation		▓	▓	▓	▓	▓	▓	▓	▓			
Armpit, leg hair			▓	▓	▓	▓	▓	▓	▓			
Adult pubic hair					▓	▓	▓	▓	▓	▓		
Full breast development					▓	▓	▓	▓	▓	▓		

study found that those who feel most different are girls who start maturing at a very young age and boys who start developing quite late.

It can help a lot to talk with your parents and let them know how you feel. If you're being teased at school about your changes or lack of changes, they may be able to help you deal with this—either by realizing what you're going through and giving you permission to shave your legs (if that's what you need to do) or by reassuring you that you're normal and loved.

Talking with your doctor can be helpful, too. Although you don't need medical help for the changes of puberty unless you have a possible problem (like not showing much, if any, development by the age of 15 or 16), checking with your doctor from time to time can help a lot. Your doctor will be able to answer any questions you and your parents have about puberty. He or she can also reassure you that you're normal and growing up in your own special way.

Time will take care of a lot of differences in growth rates between you and your friends. By your mid- to late teens, it will be hard to tell who grew up early and who started puberty later on. In time, everyone will look pretty much the same.

There will always be some individual differences, of course. Some people are naturally tall and some will always be shorter than average. Some girls will normally have larger- or smaller-than-average breasts. Some young men may never develop much or any chest hair.

These differences depend a lot on the special blend of inherited traits you got from your parents, grandparents and ancestors through centuries past. It's important to understand what's normal for your family and for your racial or ethnic background.

You're very much like your family in some ways. And you're more like your friends in other ways. That's all part of what makes you a unique person.

Once you know that you're normal, you can begin to enjoy the unique young adult you're growing to be!

How Girls Grow
and Change

What I want to know is what will it be like to change into a teenager?
How can I tell if I'm normal or not? What should I expect to happen?
Please let me know. I'm too embarrassed to ask anyone I know.
✽ JENNIFER S.

G rowing and changing is confusing at times. You don't quite look like a child or quite like an adult. In some ways, too, you may not look exactly like many of your friends. As we saw in the last chapter, people experience the changes of puberty at a wide variety of ages and in many different ways.

But wait a minute! Although you may be unique in terms of *when* certain changes happen, the actual changes happen to everyone eventually and follow certain definite patterns.

Growing into a teenager and then into an adult doesn't happen overnight, but over a period of years. The physical changes that happen will occur in stages. There are stages for just about every change you'll have—from breast development to the growth of pubic hair. And when you get your first menstrual period is tied to these other stages. In fact, you can guess, by figuring out what stage you're in with other physical changes, if you're going to be starting to menstruate soon or not.

It can really help you to feel more comfortable and *normal* when you have a clear picture of what will be happening to your body, inside and out, during the next few years.

From Girl To Woman: How It All Begins

Help! I'm scared about what's happening to me. I'm getting hair in the area between my legs, which I know is normal. But what's really gross and scary is that my lips there (is that the right word?) are growing and getting all wrinkled and awful-looking! WHAT'S THE MATTER WITH ME????? ❋ SCARED

We had a special class at school where the teacher kept using words I didn't understand. She said that they describe what's inside and out-side a woman. But I'm still confused. What exactly is a vagina? Does every girl have one? Or don't you get one until you grow up? I'm scared to ask any of my friends. They'll think I'm dumb. What was the teacher talking about? ❋ MELINDA Q.

Before you can understand the changes that are happening and will happen during the next few years, you need to understand your body.

Girls and women have special organs on the inside and outside of their bodies. All of these have been there since before they were born. Even the tiny egg cells in a girl's ovaries, the cells that will play a major role in making babies of her own some day, are already present when a baby girl is born. The difference between a baby girl, a little girl and a young woman is that her special female body parts grow and mature as her whole body grows and changes.

What are these special body parts called?

There are the *external female genitalia,* which is a name for the parts of her body that she can see in the pubic area between her legs. Then there are the *internal reproductive organs.* She can't see these, but these are very important, too, because they produce hormones that bring about many of her physical changes during puberty, cause menstruation and may, in time, enable her to have children of her own.

The whole external genital area in females is called the *vulva.* Along with reading the following descriptions, you can better understand what this is by referring to the illustrations on this page or, if you feel comfortable with the idea, looking at your own genital area.

The most obvious part of the vulva (see Fig. 3-1) are the two sets of lips that cover the other external genitalia. The outer lips are called *labia majora.* If you have reached a certain stage in puberty, these outer lips will be covered with hair. In some women, the outer lips cover the other external genitals. In other, also normal, women, the inner lips, called *labia minora,* will protrude. These inner lips may be as large or larger than the outer lips, or they may be very small. They may range in color from pink to brown, and they may be smooth or

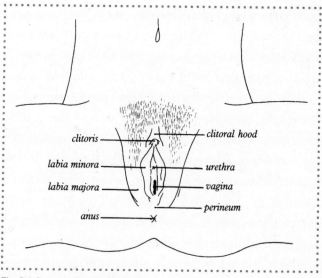

Fig. 3-1 *External Female Genitalia*

wrinkled. In her letter, Scared was describing her inner lips as strange and gross. But, in fact, they are normal in appearance.

At the point where the labia minora seem to meet, near the top of your vulva, is the *clitoris*. This is a tiny organ that is the female's equivalent to the male's penis. It is very sensitive and can play a major role in sexual arousal. The clitoris grows and becomes more sensitive and noticeable as you grow and develop.

Just below the clitoris is the *urethra*. This is the tiny opening your urine passes through. It looks like a small dimple.

The *vaginal opening* is beneath the urethra. In many girls, this opening is partially covered by the *hymen,* a thin ring of tissue. Traditionally, many people have thought that having a hymen is the sign that a girl is a virgin—that she has not had sexual intercourse. But today, we know that isn't necessarily so. Many girls are born without a hymen, and many others have their hymens stretched or torn in nonsexual ways, such as during strenuous exercise. Having a hymen or not having one are both simply variations of normal female anatomy.

The vaginal opening is important because it is the point connecting the external and internal female genitals. The *vagina* (see Fig. 3-2) is a flexible, moist passageway that leads from the vaginal opening to the *cervix,* which is the neck of the uterus. The cervix is fairly small. If you reach far back into your vagina and press on it gently, you'll find that it feels like a larger version of the tip of your nose, with a dimple in the center. This dimple is the small opening into the uterus and is called the *os.* The menstrual flow comes through the os and down the vagina on its way out of the body. And, believe it or not, this tiny opening can stretch large enough to allow a baby to pass through. But most of the time, even in adult women, this opening is very tiny.

The *uterus* (Figs. 3-2 and 3-3) is a small, muscular organ shaped like an upside-down pear. It is hollow, with a special lining of tissue inside called the *endometrium.* The interior of the uterus is usually very small, about the size of a slit, when a woman is not pregnant. When she has a baby growing in her uterus, however, this amazing

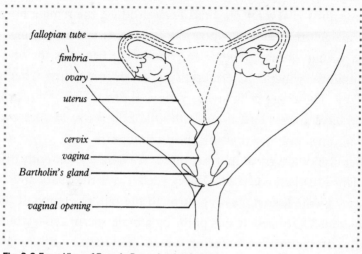

Fig. 3-2 *Front View of Female Reproductive System*

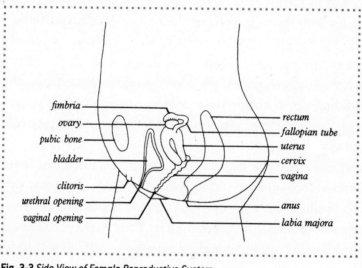

Fig. 3-3 *Side View of Female Reproductive System*

organ can expand to many times its original size. Then, after the baby is born, it will become small again.

The *fallopian tubes* extend from the top of the uterus. Near the ends of these fingerlike projections are two small organs about the size of a pea or small lima bean. These are called the *ovaries*. The ovaries are important for several reasons. They produce the female hormone called estrogen that makes it possible for you to change from a little girl to a young woman. They also contain the egg cells, or *ova*. The ova contain the genetic material that a woman contributes when making a baby. These egg cells are very tiny, about the size of a grain of salt. You have always had about 250,000 of these ova in your ovaries. But it isn't until puberty that they begin to mature.

When the ova start to mature, one is released each month from an ovary. This is called *ovulation*. The egg cell leaves the ovary and begins its journey to the uterus, passing through the fallopian tube. If the egg cell is met and fertilized at this point by a male sperm cell—which has entered the woman's body during sexual intercourse—this small collection of cells, which will grow into a baby during the next nine months, travels through the fallopian tube and into the uterus, where it attaches itself to the rich walls of the endometrium, the lining of the uterus.

If the egg isn't fertilized—and most during a woman's reproductive life are not—it disintegrates. So does the endometrial tissue that has been building up in anticipation of nourishing a fertilized egg. This blood-rich tissue is what passes out of the body as the menstrual flow each month.

But even before you begin to experience ovulation and menstruation, wonderful changes are taking place inside. As your growing body begins to produce more hormones, your ovaries and uterus grow and the lining of the uterus becomes thicker. Your vagina becomes deeper and you will notice some vaginal secretions—usually a clear-to-whitish discharge on your underwear—sometime before your first menstrual period.

Many girls worry about this discharge when they first notice it. They're afraid that they may have an infection or that something is terribly wrong. This discharge is completely normal and simply a sign that you're growing up. It's true that some infections and sexually transmitted diseases do cause discharges. But these are different. They're usually a somewhat different color (like greenish-yellow), tend to cause irritation (a burning sensation or very noticeable soreness or itching) and may have a foul odor. Your normal discharge does not. (Of course, any body secretion—from a vaginal discharge to perspiration—can develop an odor if you don't bathe and change your underwear daily.)

There are some other changes you may also notice around this time. Your sweat glands will become more active, and you will begin to perspire under your arms. Your body's oil glands will become more active, too. That means that the skin on your face, chest and back may become oily and you may develop acne (what people most often call pimples or zits).

Your Growing, Changing Breasts

Please tell me what to do. I have a sort of lump under each nipple on my chest. (I don't have real breasts yet.) Does this mean I have cancer? I saw a show on TV that said breast lumps can be cancer. Could I have breast cancer even if I don't really have breasts and am only 10 years old? That area is a little sore, too. I'm scared to tell anyone. ✳ MOLLY T.

I have really weird breasts. Truly. I half-hide in my locker when changing for gym class so no one will see them. My nipples and that area of skin around them puff out from the rest of my breast and form their own little mound on top of each breast. What causes this? Do I have some type of disease? Can a doctor do something to make my breasts look normal? Or can I do something to change them? It's really embarrassing! ✳ AMANDA G.

What Molly is describing are breast buds, the first stage of growth that developing breasts go through. (Breast buds are actually considered the second stage of breast development, with stage one being no development at all. See Figs. 3-4 to 3-8.) The breast bud occurs when the tis-

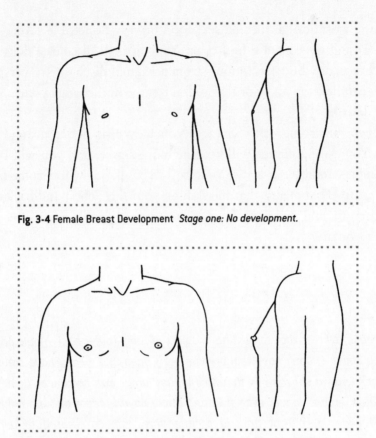

Fig. 3-4 Female Breast Development *Stage one: No development.*

Fig. 3-5 Female Breast Development *Stage two: Breast buds begin.*

sue just under the nipple elevates slightly (see Fig. 3-5). The growing breasts can be a bit tender at this stage, as Molly indicates.

During the next stage (see Fig. 3-6), the *areola,* which is the circle of skin just around the nipple, and the breast itself begin to grow quite noticeably. This is the third stage of breast development.

During the fourth stage (see Fig. 3-7), the nipple and areola form a small, separate mound that protrudes from the breast. This is what Amanda is experiencing right now. This, too, is a normal part of development.

In the fifth and final stage of breast development (see Fig. 3-8), the areola becomes, once again, a part of the main contour of the breast. The breast continues to enlarge until, finally, it is round and full.

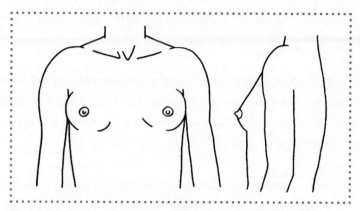

Fig. 3-6 Female Breast Development *Stage three: Breast and areola grow.*

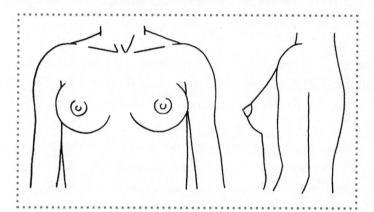

Fig. 3-7 Female Breast Development *Stage four: Nipple and areola form separate mound.*

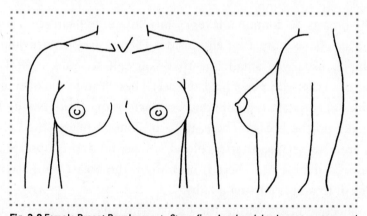

Fig. 3-8 Female Breast Development *Stage five: Areola rejoins breast contour and development is complete.*

The whole process of breast development is gradual, taking an average of four years to complete.

This probably sounds strange, but what's in breasts? Is it milk? Or fat? Or what? Are there muscles in the breasts? Can you make breasts bigger with special exercises? And what color are the nipples and the area around them supposed to be? ✳ JODIE Y.

Why do some people have little pointy breasts and others have round ones? If you have small breasts, does this mean you don't have enough female hormones? Please let me know right away because I'm worried! ✳ ELIZABETH K.

The size of your breasts tends to be inherited from your mother's side of the family or from the women on your father's side. The size and color of the areola are also inherited characteristics. The areola normally ranges in color from light pink to dark brown, depending on your complexion. Small breasts are not a sign of hormonal problems. They may be naturally smaller than average. Or they may still be developing. Your weight may have something to do with breast size, too. If you're very skinny, your breasts may be less full than average. If you're considerably overweight, fat padding may increase breast size.

The breasts do contain a layer of fat. But, as you can see from Fig. 3-9, breasts have quite a lot else inside. There are several openings in the nipple, usually a small one that you can see and several even smaller ones that you probably can't see. These lead to the openings of the milk ducts. There is a milk duct for each of the about twenty lobes that make up the breast. These, in turn, contain many small glands. There are also nerves, arteries, blood vessels, fat and lymph channels packed into the breast! There is no milk in the breast until a woman gives birth to and is nursing a baby.

Connective fibers within the breast help give it its final rounded shape. There are no muscles in the breasts, so you can't increase your

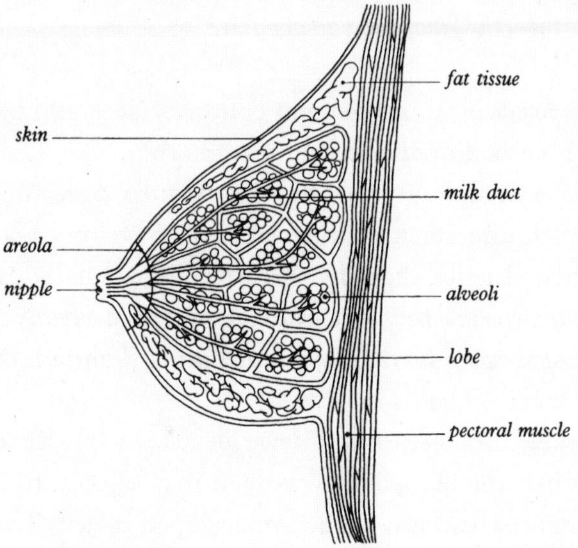

Fig. 3-9 *The Female Breast*

breast size with exercises (or with commercially advertised "bust development" devices, lotions or creams). However, there are pectoral muscles on the chest wall just beneath the breasts. Developing these muscles through weight-lifting and other exercises may lead to an increase in your all-around bust measurement (as it is measured around your torso), but it will not increase your actual breast size.

> ***I'm really upset because I have one breast that's a different size from the other. I'm 12 years old and feel like a freak! What can I do?***
> ✻ PATTI D.

> ***What does it mean if your nipples don't stand out like normal ones? Mine look like little slits. I'm scared. Does this mean I have cancer or won't be able to feed a baby if I have one?*** ✻ JOANNA A.

> ***Don't print my name. Just tell me what to do! I have some little dark hairs around the nipples of my breasts! My sister said that if I pluck***

them or try to get rid of them any other way, I'll get cancer. This hair looks just hideous! What can I do about it? ✳ WORRIED

These letters are typical of common concerns teens and preteens have about their breasts. But all three girls are normal.

Patti has a complaint many young women have: uneven breast development. Quite often, one breast will develop at a faster rate than the other. Usually, the other breast will eventually catch up. But it's important to realize that breasts rarely perfectly match one another. Most women have one breast that is slightly larger than the other.

In rare cases, one breast will never develop while the other grows normally. When this happens, a woman may choose to have plastic surgery to increase the size of the undeveloped breast. This isn't done during the growing years, however. Breast surgery is usually not performed on young women until one or both breasts have reached full development.

What Joanna is describing are called inverted nipples. These are nipples that turn inward instead of outward. This can happen in both male and female breasts and is a condition usually present from birth. It is only when a nipple has been turned out and then, later on, becomes inverted that doctors worry about a possible underlying tumor.

Sometimes, as the breast grows and develops, the enlargement of the breast tissue will cause one or both of the inverted nipples to turn out. This can also happen during breast enlargement when a woman is pregnant. Even if a woman's nipples continue to be inverted after she has had a child, she may still be able to nurse her baby with the use of special nursing shields made especially for mothers with inverted nipples who want to breast-feed their babies.

Worried, who has some hair around her nipples, has a very common concern. Getting some stray hairs around your nipples is usually not a sign that anything is wrong. It may be due to your own unique hormonal balance or your ethnic origins. Women whose ancestors

came from the Mediterranean area or the Middle East are more likely
to have more body hair than Asians or those with Nordic roots.

Only if you get hairs around your nipples *and* start developing a
lot of hair on your face along with other possibly masculine traits do
you need to check with your doctor. If it turns out that you have a hormone imbalance, you can get effective treatment for this via prescription drugs from your doctor.

Removing hair around the nipple will not harm you in any way. It's
simply a matter of choice. Some women pluck the hairs and others use
a hair removal lotion or cream (the gentle kind made for removal of
facial hair may be the best for use on the breasts). These hair removal
methods aren't permanent and have to be repeated whenever new hairs
appear—which is not a major problem once you get used to the idea.
Some women choose to have excess hair removed permanently by electrolysis. This involves a tiny electrode entering the hair follicle via a
small needle. Once there, the electrode discharges a high-speed electric
current that destroys the hair root. Electrolysis, which can be expensive, is a somewhat painful procedure. It is *extremely* important that it
be done by a qualified professional. If you're interested in electrolysis,
ask your doctor or your local medical association for suggestions and
recommendations.

> *This probably sounds dumb, but I want to know about bras. When
> should you get a bra? (Like how old should you be?) And how do you
> know what size to get? I was in a store with one of my friends yester-
> day and we looked over the boxes of bras with all kinds of strange
> numbers on them. How do you know what size to get? I mean, what
> does a 28 or 32 mean? How do you know if you are AA or A or B or C?
> Those are some of the sizes we saw. My mother says I'm too young to
> have a bra even though I have breasts already.* ✳ TAMI L.

Some women choose never to wear bras, but most American women
do. There is no particular age or stage of development when you
absolutely should or shouldn't wear a bra. It's a matter of personal

choice. If you're just starting to develop breasts, it can be a problem when you and your parents disagree about the timing for your first bra. If you have quite obvious breast development and feel uncomfortable not wearing a bra, then you really do need one. When you and your parents disagree, it's important to let them know that you feel uncomfortable not wearing a bra. The more mature you can be in discussing the matter, the more likely they will see your point of view. Or if you have very little development yet, but most of your friends are wearing bras, it may help boost your morale to get a "trainer bra," a stretchable bra made just for this stage.

How do you know what size bra to get? Bra sizes usually have a number and a letter. The number refers to the distance in inches around your torso, measured just under the breasts (see Fig. 3-10). The letter refers to the shallowness or fullness of the bra cup; this is known as the "cup size." The most common cup sizes are A, B and C. The A is for those with relatively small breasts and C is for those with fairly full, rounded breasts; those who wear a B cup fall in between. There are also some special sizes, such as AA for developing young teens and D or DD for women with much fuller than average breasts.

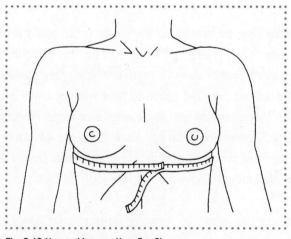

Fig. 3-10 *How to Measure Your Bra Size*

For the best fit, it is a good idea to measure yourself as the illustration shows before going shopping for a bra. Or go to a store that has a trained saleswoman who can advise you about size. She can also help you choose the best bra style for your shape of breast. Styles differ a good deal, and you may find that a particular company's 34A bra, for example, does not fit you as well as another company's bra in the same size.

If all this sounds just too embarrassing to imagine, keep in mind that such a person sells bras every day and doesn't think anything about seeing your breasts. An experienced saleswoman, in fact, has probably fitted many young girls with their first bras and will know just how to put you at ease.

If you still can't handle the idea of talking with a stranger about your breast size, seek help and advice from your mother, another older female relative or a trusted girlfriend. Keep in mind that the idea of having breasts and getting measured for a first bra can be embarrassing for you and some of your friends just because the whole experience is so new.

Older teens and adult women are so used to having breasts and buying and wearing bras that they really don't think it's such a big deal. It's all just a normal part of being a grown-up.

I'm really upset because I have something the matter with a breast! I've been wearing a bra for about a year already and everything was fine until I got this lump under my nipple. It's really sore! I'm scared to tell my mother or go to the doctor. What is it??? ✻ JILL T.

What Jill is describing is probably an adolescent nodule. This can happen even to boys and is fairly common during puberty. An adolescent nodule causes swelling under the nipple, which becomes tender and painful.

It isn't known for sure what causes these nodules, but they may be due to the increased levels of hormones at puberty. They usually disappear in time, but it may help to check with your doctor for reassurance that all is well. Girls and women do get breast lumps for a number of reasons, and it can ease your anxiety to know that your breast condition is not a sign of disease.

> *I'm 12 and have had my period for almost a year now. What I want to know is why my breasts get sore before my period. I thought I felt a lump in one of them, but when I checked again about a week later, it was gone. Am I old enough to get breast cancer? Should I go to the doctor?* ✳ KATIE C.

Most breast lumps, especially those in teenagers, tend to be benign. That means that you don't have cancer. Many girls and women have tender breasts and even some breast lumps at certain points in their menstrual cycles, usually just before their period starts.

You should tell your doctor about this so he or she can examine you at various points in your cycle and discover what kind of breast lump you may have. There are lots of different kinds. If you are having menstrual periods already and tend to get sore, lumpy breasts in the days just before your period begins, your doctor may give you some helpful suggestions. For example, some women find it helpful to cut down on salty foods in the days before menstruation is due to begin. Some women, too, have found that they have less lumpiness and pain if they cut out caffeine, a substance found in cola drinks, coffee, tea and all forms of chocolate. Your doctor will be able to advise you what might be most helpful for you.

> *How old should you be before you do breast self-examination? I heard about this on the TV news and my mother says she does it regularly, but she doesn't know whether I should be doing it already. What do you think? I'm 11½ and wear a 30A bra. I don't have any lumps (I don't think), but should I be looking for them anyway?* ✳ SHANNA W.

Although breast cancer is not especially common in preteens or teenagers, it's a good idea to make regular breast self-examination a habit. It's vital, at any age, to watch out for your health and be aware of any physical changes. If you learn what your breasts feel like now, and how and if they change with your monthly menstrual cycle, you'll be more likely to notice if anything unusual occurs later on.

How do you examine your breasts? The first step is easy: Look in the mirror. Do your breasts have any dimples? Has a nipple suddenly become inverted? Is the skin texture changing on your breast? Older women also look for changing breast contours. But when your breasts are changing and growing anyway, as yours probably are right now, changing contours are normal for you and not likely to be a sign that something is wrong.

The second part of a breast self-examination means actually feeling your breasts. You should do this at the same time each month, maybe about a week after your menstrual period is due to begin. Many women find it is easiest to examine their breasts while they shower or bathe or while lying in bed.

This second part of your breast self-exam is illustrated in Figs. 3-11 to 3-14. Here is what you need to do:

First, touch every part of your breast, working from the outer contours to the nipple area in a gentle, circular, clockwise motion. Feel for any lumps or thickening of breast tissue.

Then repeat the exam in another position. If you were standing during the first, lie down. Extend your right arm over your head. With your left hand, repeat the circular examination of your right breast. Then switch arms. Extend your left arm over your head and use your right hand to examine your left breast.

If you notice anything unusual, check with your doctor. Because breast cancer is quite rare in teenagers, any lumps or other unusual breast symptoms are likely to be a sign of a minor rather than major problem, but only your doctor can tell you this.

Getting into the habit of taking a few minutes each month to examine your breasts is a healthful choice that could someday even save your life!

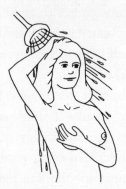

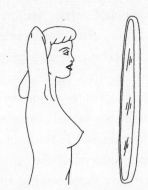

Fig. 3-11 Breast Self-Examination
Check your breasts for any thickening or lumps.

Fig. 3-12 Breast Self-Examination
Raise your arms and look in the mirror for changes in contour, skin texture or color.

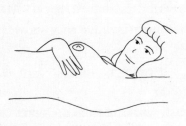

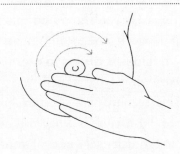

Fig. 3-13 Breast Self-Examination
Lie down and repeat examination.

Fig. 3-14 Breast Self-Examination
Always use a circular, clockwise motion.

Pubic Hair Development

Is it normal if you have pubic hair that's straight instead of curly and if there isn't very much of it? Answer me quick! ✻ LEIGH Y.

I just started seventh grade and we have to undress for gym in front of each other. I notice that everyone has different amounts of hair on their private parts. Will everyone look more alike when we get older, or will we always look so different from each other? ✻ KIM B.

Even though there can be normal ethnic differences in pubic hair—some Asians or Asian Americans, for example, tend to have less extensive pubic hair patterns—most people grow up to look pretty much alike.

What makes preteens and teens look so different from each other is the fact that there are some very different stages of pubic hair development that everyone passes through on the way to maturity.

Pubic hair, which usually appears sometime after breast development has begun, starts off straight and fine in texture and there isn't much of it (see Figs. 3-15 and 3-16).

Next, it begins to darken, coarsen and spread a little higher up in the pubic area (Fig. 3-17).

In the next stage of development, the hair begins to look like an adult's, both in texture and in its triangular growth pattern. But it covers a more limited area than an adult's pubic hair does (Fig. 3-18).

During the final stage of pubic hair development, the full adult triangular pattern is established. This last stage can occur any time between the ages of 12 and 19, depending on when physical development begins (Fig. 3-19).

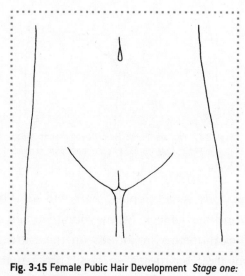

Fig. 3-15 Female Pubic Hair Development *Stage one: No pubic hair.*

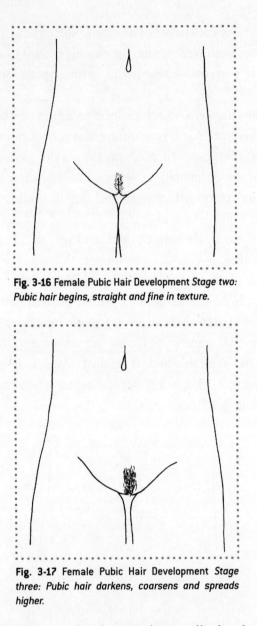

Fig. 3-16 Female Pubic Hair Development *Stage two: Pubic hair begins, straight and fine in texture.*

Fig. 3-17 Female Pubic Hair Development *Stage three: Pubic hair darkens, coarsens and spreads higher.*

(While pubic hair is developing, hair will also begin to appear under the arms and on the legs. Many young women choose to shave or use hair removal creams or lotions on these areas to keep them smooth and hair-free, but doing so is simply a matter of personal choice.)

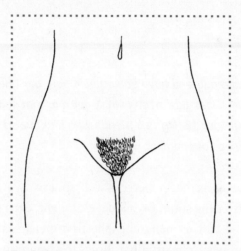

Fig. 3-18 Female Pubic Hair Development *Stage four: Pubic hair has adult texture and shape, but covers a smaller area.*

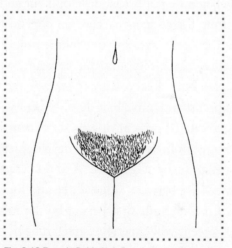

Fig. 3-19 Female Pubic Hair Development *Stage five: Full adult pubic hair pattern.*

Menstruation

I wear a bra already and have some pubic hair, but I haven't had my first period yet. Does this mean I won't get it or that something is the matter? I'm almost 12. My two friends who look pretty much like me have their periods already! ✳ CHRISTY A.

Christy has some signs that puberty is well underway. And she will probably start menstruating soon. Breast development, even if it is very slight, will always come before menarche, the first menstrual period. Studies have shown that menarche usually follows the beginning of breast development by two to three years. However, girls who begin breast development at the earlier range of normal—at age 8 or 9—may have a shorter time between the beginning of breast development and menarche.

The normal time for your menarche can depend a lot on your heritage. Looking at menarche ages of your mother, older sisters, aunts and other female relatives can give you a clue to your own possible starting age. You can also tell how close you are to starting menstruation by finding what stage of breast and pubic hair development you're in. According to recent studies, about 10 percent of girls start menstruating when they are in the second stage of breast/pubic hair development. Another 20 percent have their menarche by stage three. And 60 percent more will begin their periods somewhere between stages three and four. So you have a 90 percent chance of having your first period by the time you reach stage four. The last 10 percent will experience menarche by stage five.

Another way you can tell that menstruation is near is by looking at your growth rate. During these years, your body is growing taller and changing shape quickly (see Figs. 2-5 to 2-8). It's likely that your menarche will occur about six months after you have reached the peak of your growth spurt and weight gain.

Many girls get upset about this weight gain and start dieting at this time. But it's important to know that mature women *need* a certain level of body fat in order to menstruate normally.

Studies have shown that, in order to start menstruating and have regular monthly periods, a woman needs to maintain a weight that allows fat to comprise 17 to 22 percent of her total body weight. This balance of fat helps stimulate the hormone production that regulates menstruation. If your level of body fat falls below this percentage, you may have a delayed menarche.

The girls most likely to have delayed menarche are those with low body weight: chronic dieters, competitive runners, gymnasts and serious ballet dancers.

In a study of young New York–based ballet dancers, Dr. Jeanne Brooks-Gunn, a scientist famous for her research on menstruation, compared the weights and menarche ages of dancers who were all about the same height, 5'4". Those with the lowest average weight—105 pounds—tended to be the latest in starting their periods. But the dancers who were only a little underweight—115 pounds—tended to experience menarche at about the same time as nondancers who weighed an average of 125 pounds. These latter two groups began to menstruate close to the average age, at around 12 or 13. Studies show that exercise may be less of a factor in the onset of menstruation than weight or diet. For example, competitive swimmers may train just as hard as gymnasts, runners or dancers, but the requirement for lower weight is not nearly as strict in their sport.

So if you're very active in a demanding sport and have a low fat level or if you are extremely thin due to constant dieting, you may experience menarche considerably later than your female relatives and friends.

Could you tell me what menstruation is for and why it happens? I can't figure out what's good about it. My mom calls it "the curse." She hates having her periods. It makes me feel bad because I just started menstruating three months ago and everything I read tells me that I'll probably have periods for thirty or forty more years! ❋ DEBI U.

I hear people talk about menstrual periods. And then they say menstrual cycle. Are these the same thing? I'm embarrassed to ask anyone directly because I don't want them to think I'm stupid or something. ❋ MISSY R.

Now that I've had my first period, I'm getting all sorts of "wonderful" advice. My grandma told me that I shouldn't wash my hair or take a bath during my period. I don't think that's right. My mother says I shouldn't exercise during my period and that makes me upset because I really love sports and am on my school's volleyball team. What if I get my period just before a big game? What should I do?
✳ MARY-THERESA M.

I don't have my period yet, but I worry about it all the time. The reason I worry is because . . . what if I get it at school or when I'm at a friend's house? What would I do? What could I say to people? ✳ JAMIE L.

As these letters show, girls have a lot of questions and uncertainties about menstruation as they go through puberty.

Menstruation is a very healthy, normal process experienced by most women—except during pregnancy—from puberty through menopause, which usually occurs in the late forties or early fifties. (Menopause is the end of the female's reproductive capacity, when she stops having menstrual periods.)

Even though some women call it "the curse" or think that having your period means you can't be active or follow your normal routines—like bathing or washing your hair—menstruation is *not* a curse, an illness or a negative happening. In fact, it is a sign that you're healthy and that your growing or grown-up body is functioning just the way it should!

Until recently, though, there were a lot of myths and superstitions about menstruation and little bits of these still hang on in some people's minds. Through the centuries, it was thought that menstruation was mysterious because it involved bleeding with no injury. People couldn't understand this and began to think that women either had scary, mystical powers or that they were unclean.

Today we know the truth about menstruation. We know it is a normal body function that happens for a very good reason. What is this reason?

Every month your body begins to prepare itself for a possible pregnancy. As we have seen earlier, an egg cell ripens in your ovary and is released into the fallopian tube to journey down into the uterus (Fig. 3-20). While the egg is on its way, the uterus begins preparing itself to nourish a possible baby. The blood vessels in the uterus swell, and the endometrium, the lining of the uterus, begins to thicken until it is about twice its normal size (Fig. 3-21). It is here in the blood-rich endometrium that the egg, if it is fertilized by the male sperm as the result of sexual intercourse, will attach itself and begin to develop into a baby.

Most of the time, however, the egg will *not* be fertilized, so there isn't any use for all that nourishing tissue in your uterus. So your body sends a message to the swollen blood vessels to start shrinking. Over a period of days, they do, emptying their small storage of blood into the uterus in little drops (Fig. 3-22). At the same time, the thickened endometrium begins to break up and fall away. This mixture of tissue and blood then flows down through the uterus and vagina and passes out of your body. This whole process is called menstruation.

The menstrual *period* is the time when the menstrual flow is actually leaving your body. This will usually last from three to seven days. Even though it may look as if you're losing a lot of blood, you really aren't. Most women lose about 2 to 4 ounces of blood per period. That's half a cup at the most. And that isn't so much when you realize that you have 120 ounces of blood in your body and that this supply is constantly being replaced with fresh, new blood.

The menstrual *cycle* is a term that refers to everything that happens inside your body during the entire month, not just during the days you actually lose blood.

Your period is the first phase of your cycle. During the second phase, your body begins to produce more estrogen, a hormone that causes the endometrium to start growing again. During the third phase (see Fig. 3-20), an egg is released from your ovary. This is called ovulation. During the fourth phase, your body produces progesterone, another hormone, as well as estrogen. This causes the endometrium to keep thickening. Then, if the egg is not fertilized through intercourse, hormone levels drop sharply and the extra-thick lining is shed. At this

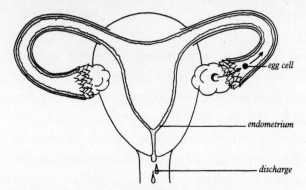

Fig. 3-20 The Menstrual Cycle: Ovulation *The ripened egg leaves the ovary and enters the fallopian tube. Often, a woman's clear vaginal discharge increases at this time.*

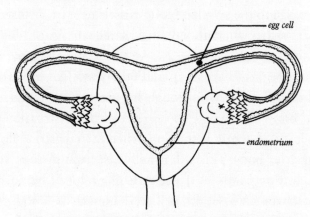

Fig. 3-21 The Menstrual Cycle: The Endometrium Grows *The uterine lining builds up in preparation for a possible fertilized egg.*

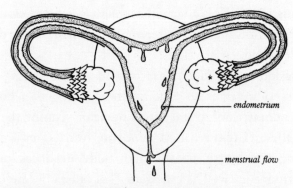

Fig. 3-22 The Menstrual Cycle: Menstruation *If the egg is not fertilized, it disintegrates. The endometrium breaks up and is released from the body as the menstrual flow.*

point you get your period again: The lining, mixed with a small amount of blood, flows out of your body through the uterus and vagina.

The whole menstrual cycle takes an average of 28 days to complete. However, some normal women have cycles that are longer or shorter. And some girls, who are just beginning to menstruate, may have very irregular periods during the first year or two after menarche. During this time, it is not uncommon for a girl to go two or three months between periods; others may menstruate as often as every two weeks for a while. Stress or illness can also cause you to miss a period every now and then. (We'll be telling you a lot more about menstrual problems—including irregular periods, premenstrual symptoms and cramps—in Chapter Nine.)

Lots of girls worry about having their first menstrual periods while away from home. If you show signs of being very close to having your first period (by having a lot of other signs of puberty), you might prepare by carrying a packaged mini-pad in your purse or making sure you have enough change to buy a tampon or sanitary pad from a restroom vending machine. If you're at a friend's house for a visit, tell your friend and, possibly, her mother or older sister. They will probably have some supplies you can use. If you get your first period at school and aren't prepared in advance, your school nurse is likely to have supplies of pads in her office. Or you can tell your teacher, who will be able to help you.

Keep in mind that your first period usually doesn't start with a big gush of blood. You'll probably feel a little wetness or notice a few spots on your underwear. So no one is going to notice you just got your period.

Having your period, whether it's your first or not, really isn't something to be embarrassed about. But many young girls do feel extremely self-conscious at such times. Studies by Dr. Jeanne Brooks-Gunn have found that it's quite common for girls to be very shy when it comes to talking about their periods around the time of menarche and for about a year or so afterward. This is probably because the whole idea of growing up and beginning to menstruate is so new to you and to your friends. When it becomes a more routine part of your life and you get used to it, you'll find that you probably won't feel so embarrassed about the whole subject. In the meantime, it may help to keep in mind that most people will not know you have your period unless you tell them. With the convenient sanitary protection available today, your menstruation is not obvious to those around you.

Once your periods are well established, you can pretty accurately predict when you'll get your next period and so be prepared for it. Counting the first day of bleeding as day one, keep track of how many days come in between that and your next period. If, for example, your next-to-last period began on December 1 and the period after that started December 29, you have a 28-day cycle. By counting 28 days from the first day of your last period, you can tell which day your next period is likely to start. Some girls carry pads or tampons with them to school when the next period is expected, and some even wear mini-pads on the day their period is due to start if it's a school day or an especially active day away from home.

So once again: *Menstruation is a good, healthy, natural process.* It doesn't have to interfere with your life at all. In fact, researchers have found that women who are fit and active tend to have fewer problems with menstrual cramps than other women. You can participate in sports, bathe, wash your hair and do anything else you enjoy doing whether or not you have your period. Menstruation is just a part of life. It doesn't have to slow down your normal life for several days or a week each month!

Could you tell me whether it's better to use tampons or pads? I like to swim, so I'd really like to use tampons, but my mother is against it because she says I'm too young (12) and she says tampons can give you a terrible disease. Is this true? I know some of my friends use tampons and none of them seem sick. What's the truth about tampons? ✳ BECKY N.

There are so many different types of pads around that I get confused. What are the best ones to use when you have only recently started your periods? ✳ MELISSA Y.

It's really a matter of personal choice whether you use tampons (rolled cylinders of cotton and other material), which are inserted into your vagina to catch the menstrual flow before it leaves your body, or sanitary pads, made of absorbent material with adhesive backing that you can stick to your underwear.

Some girls who are active in sports, especially swimming, prefer tampons—either during these activities or throughout their menstrual period. Others use tampons and pads, wearing tampons during the day and pads at night. Still others prefer to use pads all the time, or tampons all the time.

If you prefer pads, all the varieties can be confusing (see Fig. 3-23). There are many different kinds and absorbencies. The thicker, larger pads are for use during the days of your period when bleeding is heavier. These are usually called super- or maxi-pads. Mini-pads, which are smaller, may be used during the days when your flow is light. Some girls wear panty shields or liners, very thin pads, on the days when they expect to get their periods, just so they won't get spots on their underwear. Of course, you don't have to use all of these different kinds. Try a variety and see what seems right for you.

Tampons also come in a variety of absorbencies and sizes—from junior or slender sizes (especially convenient for young girls) to regular or super-absorbent varieties. Tampons can be safe and convenient. They cannot get lost in your body because there is no place for them to go. (The opening of the cervix, at the upper end of your vagina, is much too tiny for a tampon to fit through!) And they cannot cause you not to be a virgin anymore; only having sexual intercourse will make a girl a nonvirgin. However, it's important to know that tampons *have* been associated with toxic shock syndrome.

Toxic shock syndrome (TSS) is a very rare disease that has been around for years, but it was first linked with tampon use in 1978. It is caused by a bacterium that lives on the skin and in body cavities and that usually causes no problems. However, in some circumstances, such as when blood is collected and held by a surgical dressing or tampon, the bacterium may produce a toxin known as TSST-1. Toxic

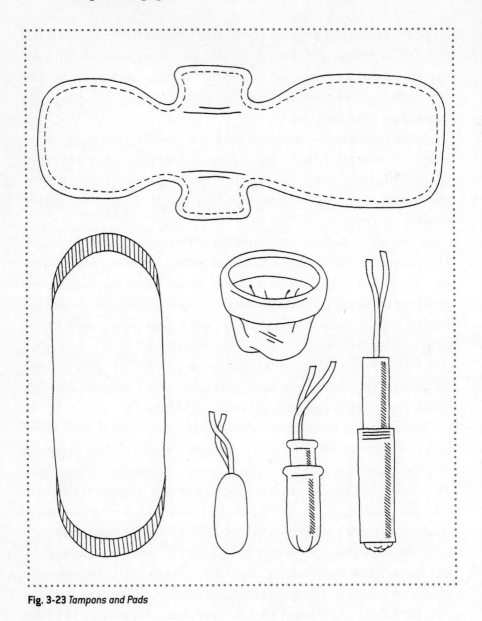

Fig. 3-23 *Tampons and Pads*

shock syndrome *usually* doesn't occur even then because most people are immune to this toxin. But young women under 25 may be somewhat less immune and more likely to develop the disease.

Toxic shock syndrome usually starts with symptoms such as a high fever (more than 102°), vomiting, diarrhea, light-headedness, aching muscles, headache and a sunburnlike rash that often develops on the hands and soles of the feet. If you have such symptoms, especially during menstruation, remove your tampon immediately and see your doctor at once! If left untreated, TSS can be fatal. These days, the fatality rate is about 3 percent, but early treatment is vital nevertheless.

Even if you use tampons all through your period, you're unlikely to get toxic shock syndrome. However, the way you use tampons can increase or decrease your chances of getting this disease.

How can you safeguard your health if you choose to wear tampons?

■ Wash your hands *before* inserting a new tampon.

■ Use tampons that are *not* highly absorbent and change them often, at least every three to four hours even when your flow is light.

■ Switch to a pad at bedtime; because you're sleeping, there will be a long interval between changes.

■ If you use a tampon that doesn't have an inserter, be careful not to scratch your vaginal wall with a fingernail. Or if the tampon has an inserter—especially one with a plastic, petal-shaped end—take care not to scratch your vaginal walls with the edges or end of the inserter. Small tears in the vaginal wall can allow bacteria and toxins to enter your bloodstream.

■ Use a pad or mini-pad instead of a tampon during the days when your period is tapering off and your flow is very light.

Most women can and do use tampons without having any health problems. But it makes sense to take a few precautions to reduce your risks even more. By using tampons wisely, you can enjoy their convenience *and* safeguard your health.

There is a new sanitary protection product out that is quite different from either tampons or pads. It is the Instead Softcup that is inserted into the vagina and catches the menstrual flow. Some young teens who just can't get used to tampons may find the Softcup a bit of a challenge to insert properly. However, if you're willing to keep trying, this product might give you a new form of convenience. If you decide to try it, please note that this should not be kept in place longer than twelve hours and a cup should *not* be reused. To do so might cause a vaginal infection.

> *What does it mean if you've had your period for over a year and then stop having it? I missed my period last month and am late getting it this month. I know I couldn't be pregnant because I don't even have a boyfriend. I'm really scared that something serious is wrong. What's the matter with me??* ✳ MARCY W.

What Marcy is describing is a condition called *secondary amenorrhea*. This means that menstrual periods come to a stop after a girl has experienced menarche.

Pregnancy is the most common cause for secondary amenorrhea among teenagers. But secondary amenorrhea may occur for a number of other reasons, too. A lot of stress in your life—like a death in the family or your parents' divorce—could cause you to skip a period or two. Moving or starting to go to a new school can also be stressful and might put a stop to your periods temporarily.

If you've had a major weight change, especially a significant weight loss, you may stop menstruating for a while. This is especially true if you have been dieting severely and are now considerably below the weight normal for your height or if you are a serious dancer or athlete with very little body fat.

The use of drugs, especially tranquilizers (downers), can also cause you to skip periods. And there are medical conditions, too, like ovarian cysts, that can disrupt your menstrual periods.

If you have missed more than one period, check with your doctor to make sure you don't have a medical condition that could be affecting your periods. After examining you, your physician will be able to make some recommendations. Occasionally, a doctor will prescribe the drug Provera to regulate the menstrual cycle for a few months until it is well established again. He or she may reassure you that your periods will probably start up again as soon as your emotional crisis has passed or when you gain a little weight and reach a fairly normal level of body fat. Keep in mind, if you're a weight-conscious athlete or dancer, that your weight gain may only have to be a few pounds to bring back your regular periods.

Keep in mind, too, that if you've been menstruating for a relatively short time—a year or less—skipping a period here and there is quite common and no cause for alarm. Of course, if a girl is sexually active—having sexual intercourse—a missed period could mean pregnancy. Whenever that may be a possibility, it's important to check with a physician right away.

Many girls wonder if they really need to have periods during the years when they aren't planning to have children anyway. There are no easy answers to this. Some experts feel that not having your period over a long period of time can cause lowered levels of the hormone estrogen and, quite possibly, result in the loss of calcium, resulting in bone weakness. Others are not convinced that secondary amenorrhea, especially when it is linked to heavy exercise, is necessarily harmful.

Until more is known about the long-term effects of prolonged secondary amenorrhea, it's a good idea to see your doctor if you've been having regular periods for more than a year and then miss more than one menstrual period consecutively.

Living With Your Growing, Changing Body

The many changes you're experiencing right now may make you feel awkward and embarrassed at times. But as you get used to your changing body, you'll begin to feel more comfortable with it.

It's important to know, like and take good care of your changing body. Feeling good about yourself physically will help you to feel better in general about growing up and about becoming a young woman.

You don't have to be as pretty as a model or as skinny as your best friend or wear a certain bra size to be a uniquely beautiful person. You don't have to have lots of boyfriends—or even one—to be a wonderful, worthwhile person. And it's fine to be different in certain ways—from developing at your own rate to having your own individual style of looking or thinking or feeling.

Accepting the way you're like your friends and different from your friends can help you grow in confidence. Welcoming instead of dreading your body's growth and changes can help you adjust to and enjoy your exciting young adulthood. And when you feel good about yourself as a woman, you'll find that other people will accept you as you are—as a unique, likable, lovable person!

4

How Boys Grow
and Change

My parents have told me all kinds of things about how babies are made, but they haven't said anything to me about how my body is supposed to change. So how will I know if I'm normal or not? How will I know what to expect? ✳ PAUL R.

When adults tell you the "facts of life," it's not unusual for them to skip over many of the facts about your body changes during puberty. Some think it isn't necessary, that somehow you know everything you need to know already. And some aren't sure what to tell you. There are so many changes and so many ways of being normal during this time.

Your physical changes during the next few years will bring many new experiences. Sometimes you'll be happy to see yourself growing taller and stronger. Sometimes you may feel awkward and embarrassed by your changing body. And other times, you may simply wonder what's going on!

Your growing-up experience will be totally unique in some ways. But in other ways, you and your friends will all be going through many of the same experiences in the next few years. You're normal, you're not so different—and you're not alone!

Becoming a teenager and then a young adult isn't something that happens all at once. Your physical changes will happen in stages. There are stages for most of the changes you'll have—from penis and testicle growth to the development of pubic hair. As you read through this chapter and study the illustrations showing these changes, you will see that, whatever stage you're in, you're following a *normal* pattern.

Knowing that you're normal can make living through all these changes a lot easier. It also helps to have a clear picture of what will be happening to your body, inside and out, during the next few years.

From Boy To Man: How It All Begins

Is it true that boys have sex organs inside their bodies besides having them outside? Or is that just another fib my friend Larry made up? ✳ KEVIN H.

I'm upset because I just started junior high and we have to take showers in this big, open shower after gym class. I haven't developed as much as a lot of the guys and my penis is a lot smaller than most. It makes me not want to go to gym class anymore. Can I get a letter from a doctor excusing me from gym because I'm not as developed as the others? And, most important, does this mean I'll always have a much smaller penis than everyone I know? ✳ STEVE K.

Is it normal to have your balls grow but for your penis to stay the same size? It really looks weird! Will my penis grow later or is something wrong with me? ✳ PAUL Y.

Knowing all about your reproductive system—the parts you can easily see and the ones you can't—can help you better understand some of your soon-to-happen physical changes.

Your outside—or external—sex organs are the *penis* and the *scrotum*. That's probably not news to you. But there are some things you may not have heard about these important organs.

For example, some people think that the penis is just a sort of skin-covered tube. Some think that, because it sometimes gets stiff, it has a bone in it. In fact, the penis does not have a bone and it isn't some sort of hollow tube.

The penis is made up of spongy tissues with lots of large blood vessels interlaced with them. When the penis gets stiff—a process called *erection*—it is because these blood vessels have expanded, bringing more blood into the penis. There are special valves in these vessels that keep this blood trapped in the penis for a while. The soft tissues of the penis expand and become hard. If you look at the illustration (Fig. 4-1), you will see how different an erect penis looks from a nonerect (called flaccid) penis. When the erect penis expands in size and lifts up, the scrotum underneath becomes tighter and more rounded and rises, too.

Boys get erections for lots of reasons. Thinking about sex or being

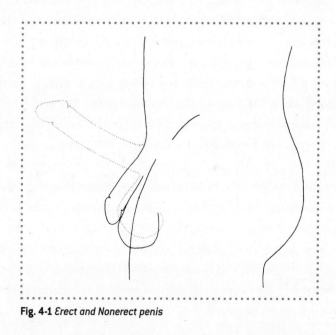

Fig. 4-1 *Erect and Nonerect penis*

with a girl you like can do it. But you can also get an erection for no special reason—just riding in a car or bus or sitting in class. It doesn't even matter what you're thinking. You may be thinking of homework or a football game or nothing in particular and *still* get an erection. If this happens to you and you're feeling really embarrassed, it may help to remember that erections happen to every male and they aren't nearly as noticeable to others as you may think.

It's very common for boys who are going through physical changes to worry about their penis size and about looking different from other boys. It may be comforting to remember that there *is* a lot of normal variation in size.

If you haven't yet begun to develop, your penis will, quite naturally, be smaller than that of a friend or classmate who is well into puberty. Also, if you're in one of the earlier stages of puberty, it is very normal for your scrotum and testicles to grow noticeably some time before your penis begins its growth.

Even among mature males, there is a wide variation in *normal* penis sizes. The average *adult* male's penis is 3 to 4 inches long and 1¼ inches in diameter in the flaccid state. But it's also normal to have a penis that is somewhat smaller or larger than average. And when the penis is erect, the size differences among men are much less noticeable.

Another difference that many boys worry about while taking after-gym showers together is that some boys have a piece of skin partially or completely covering the head of the penis (see Figs. 4-2 and 4-3). This is called the *foreskin* and is present in all male babies when they are born. Many boys have this foreskin cut back in a procedure called circumcision. All baby boys born into the Jewish faith are circumcised as part of a religious ritual soon after birth. And many other hospital-born male babies are circumcised by a physician before they leave the hospital if that's what their parents choose. Although a circumcised penis and an uncircumcised penis may look somewhat different (see the illustrations), they function in exactly the same way. Neither way to be is better than the other; it's simply a matter of religious or cultural choice.

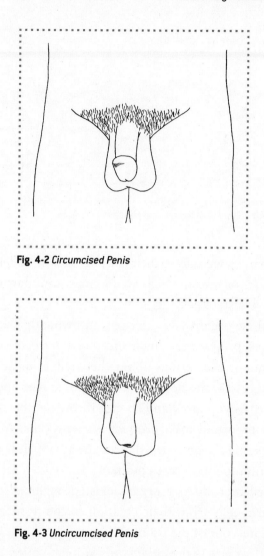

Fig. 4-2 *Circumcised Penis*

Fig. 4-3 *Uncircumcised Penis*

If you are uncircumcised, however, it's important to wash your penis thoroughly whenever you shower or bathe. A foul-smelling substance called smegma can collect under the foreskin if the penis is not washed daily. And some boys who don't practice good daily hygiene can get irritating infections of the tip, or glans, of the penis or have difficulty retracting the foreskin. To avoid such problems, pull your foreskin back and wash the head of your penis carefully while you're bathing.

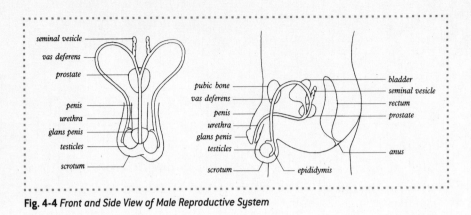

Fig. 4-4 *Front and Side View of Male Reproductive System*

The scrotum, as we said earlier, is a sac of skin under the penis. It holds the *testicles* or testes, which are an important part of your internal reproductive system (see Fig. 4-4).

What are these organs you can't see, and what do they do?

The testicles produce the male hormone *testosterone*. It is this important hormone that brings about the changes of adolescence for boys—genital growth, the development of pubic hair and the deepening of the voice. As you grow and change through puberty, the testicles begin another important task: producing sperm cells. A sperm cell, if united with a woman's egg cell, will produce a baby. It is the male's genetic contribution to any future children.

The internal reproductive organs exist to make, store and transport these sperm cells from their creation in the testicles to the time they are ejaculated out of the tip of the penis.

For example, there is the *epididymis,* a long, coiled canal that lies over each testicle. The sperm cells travel through these canals when they first leave the testicles. Then they go on to the *vas deferens,* which is a shorter continuation of the epididymis. By now, they have traveled from the scrotum into the abdomen, around in back of the bladder and into the *seminal vesicles,* which form an *ejaculatory duct* where the sperm are stored.

The *prostate gland* is right next to the bottom of the bladder. This gland, which increases dramatically in size when you reach puberty, produces a special fluid. This sticky, white substance, combined with fluids from the seminal vesicles, carries the sperm cells from the body. This is called *seminal fluid*.

But seminal fluid isn't the only secretion your internal sex organs make. In the *urethra*, a passageway in the penis that can carry both seminal fluid and urine (but never at the same time, because a valve connecting your bladder and your urethra automatically closes when seminal fluid and sperm cells are passing through the urethra), there are two tiny glands on either side that also produce a fluid. These are called *bulbourethral glands* or *Cowper's glands*. They produce a clear, sticky substance when a man is sexually excited. This fluid is thought to coat the urethra to help the passage of sperm out of the penis.

What does it mean when fluid comes out of your penis when you're sleeping? I know I didn't wet the bed, but something happened and I'm not sure what. Does this mean something is wrong with me? I hope I don't have to see a doctor because I hate to think of telling my mom why I want to go. ✳ KYLE C.

How many sperm does a man usually have? Can you use them all up before you're old enough to get married and then not be able to have children? ✳ SCOTT R.

Sperm and seminal fluid are ejected from the penis in a process called *ejaculation* (see Fig. 4-5). This can happen in several ways: when a male is having sex, is sexually excited or is asleep.

Ejaculation that occurs while you are asleep is called a *nocturnal emission* or "wet dream." Wet dreams are perfectly normal. They are simply your body's way of making room in your seminal vesicles for newer sperm cells. Wet dreams can happen to any male but are most common in adolescent boys who are not yet sexually active in any way.

Once you've reached puberty and your testicles begin to produce sperm cells, this process goes on continuously for the rest of your life. So it isn't really possible to run out of sperm, no matter how often you

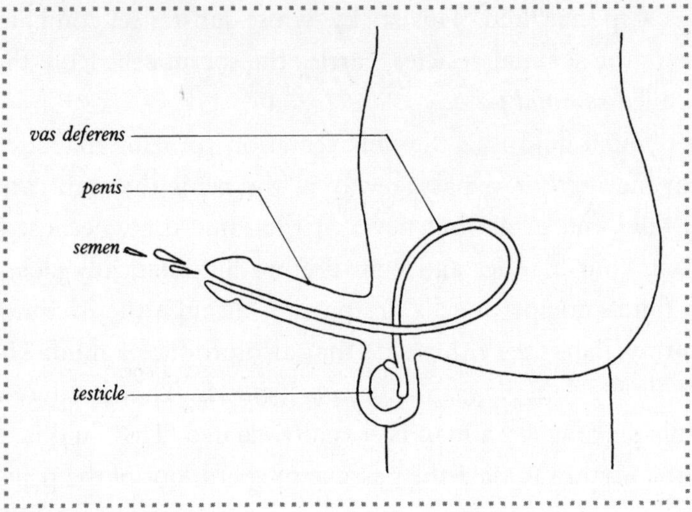

Fig. 4-5 *Ejaculation*

ejaculate. You're likely to produce billions of sperm in your lifetime. Each ejaculation amounts to only about a teaspoon of fluid. But within that small amount are about 400 million sperm cells!

Growing In Stages

> ***The last time I went to the doctor's for an exam, he said I was in the "second stage" of development. WHAT DOES THAT MEAN??? I was too embarrassed to ask. How many stages are there? How can a doctor tell just by looking at you undressed what stage you're in?***
>
> ✲ MARK S.

Your body grows and changes in distinct stages. Your shape changes gradually—from that of a child to that of a more muscular, broad-shouldered young man—as puberty progresses. Along with this change of shape come other changes: genital growth, pubic hair and skin and voice changes. As you can see from the illustrations, each stage has its own distinctive patterns. We talked about these a bit in Chapter Two,

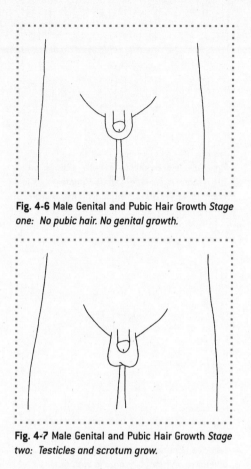

Fig. 4-6 Male Genital and Pubic Hair Growth *Stage one: No pubic hair. No genital growth.*

Fig. 4-7 Male Genital and Pubic Hair Growth *Stage two: Testicles and scrotum grow.*

but now that you know more about your body, let's review them again (see Figs. 4-6 to 4-10).

In stage one, it doesn't look like anything is happening. But inside, when you are perhaps 8 to 10 years old, hormones are becoming more active. Your testicles are beginning to mature and, late in the first stage, you may start a period of rapid growth.

In stage two, which can happen anywhere from the ages of 9 to 15, with 12 or 13 being average, you grow taller and your shape begins to change noticeably. You'll develop a somewhat more muscular look. Your testicles and scrotum grow, but your penis seems to stay about the same. You may develop a little pubic hair at the base of your penis. It's likely to be very fine and straight at this point.

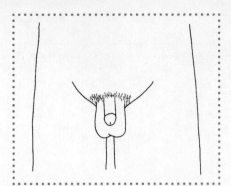

Fig. 4-8 Male Genital and Pubic Hair Growth
Stage three: Pubic hair is sparse; penis grows in length; testicles and scrotum continue to grow.

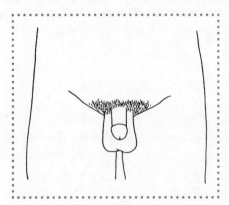

Fig. 4-9 Male Genital and Pubic Hair Growth
Stage four: Penis grows in width; scrotum and testicles continue to grow. Pubic hair coarsens and takes on triangular growth pattern.

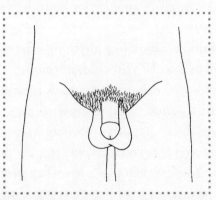

Fig. 4-10 Male Genital and Pubic Hair Growth
Stage five: Genitals and pubic hair are adult in appearance.

In stage three, which occurs between the ages of 11 and 16, but usually around 13 or 14, your testicles and scrotum continue to grow. Your penis begins to grow, too. But at this stage, it will grow mostly in length rather than width. Your pubic hair becomes darker and coarse and spreads to a wider area. Your voice is beginning to deepen as your larynx enlarges. You're still getting taller, and your shape is looking more and more like that of a grown man: broad shoulders, slim hips and more muscles. You may also have the first traces of hair on your upper lip.

In stage four, which happens between the ages of 11 and 17, with 14 or 15 as the average, your penis will grow in width as well as length. Your scrotum and testicles are also still growing. Your pubic hair has taken on an inverted triangle pattern much like an adult's, except that it covers a smaller area. It is in stage four that your testicles will begin to produce sperm cells and you will have your first ejaculation. Your voice is getting deeper and your skin oily (acne may develop at this stage). Underarm hair begins to grow, and you may have some hair growth on your chin as well.

When you reach stage five, sometime between 14 and 18, with 16 as the average, you'll be shaving and your physique will have become that of a mature male. Your genitals and pubic hair are also adult in appearance. You'll grow more body hair on your legs and arms, on your stomach and, perhaps, on your chest. Your growth is slowing down a lot, although some young men continue to grow and develop more body hair into their late teens and early twenties.

I was reading something yesterday about how boys can get cancer in the balls and how you should check yourself regularly like women are supposed to check their breasts for cancer. My question is: Should I be doing this now? I'm 11 years old. How do you do it, and what do you look for? ✳ JASON N.

Testicular cancer is one of the most common cancers in males between the ages of 15 and 35. Although Jason is a bit younger than that, it is not too early for him to be aware of how his testicles feel normally and to do regular self-exams.

Examining your testicles is an important health safeguard. Testicular cancer occurs in about 5,000 men a year. With early detection, the most common form of this disease is almost 100 percent curable and the 5-year survival rate for *all* forms of testicular cancer is about 68 percent.

Ideally, you should do your self-exam once a month, after a warm bath or shower so that your scrotum will be relaxed. Gently roll each testicle between the thumbs and fingers of both hands (see Fig. 4-11). A normal testicle feels smooth, somewhat like a hard-boiled egg. If you notice any lumps *besides* the two testicles or any unusual swelling, do see your doctor right away.

What's a jockstrap? Why do I need one? I have to get one when I start junior high. Could I get one by myself, or does my mother have to be there? (My parents are divorced and my dad lives in another state and I never see him.) How do I know what size to get—or are there sizes? What if there aren't any small enough to fit me (I'm not very developed yet) and the coach gets mad because I don't have one? How small can you be and still get a jockstrap? ✳ WORRIED

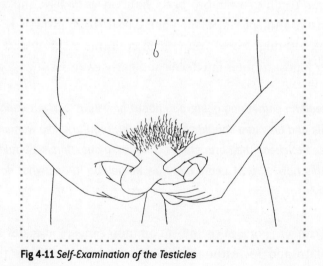

Fig 4-11 *Self-Examination of the Testicles*

Athletic supporters, also called jockstraps, are worn to support and protect the testicles during rigorous sports. The supporter keeps the testicles close to the body, making them less vulnerable to injury.

Where can you get an athletic supporter? They're sold in many places, including drugstores and sporting goods shops. You could buy one on your own or with a parent or friend. It isn't something you have to be fitted or measured for in the store. If you know your size in advance, you can just pick the right size and buy it just like that.

How do you know what size to get? That's something a *lot* of boys worry about. They think that the size of the jockstrap has to do with the size of their penis and testicles. Wrong! The size of the athletic supporter is keyed to your *waist* size. Measure your waist with a tape measure at home and then you'll have a better idea about the right size athletic supporter to get.

Some manufacturers make youth-size athletic supporters, with Regular fitting waist sizes 29 to 36 inches and Small for those with 20- to 28-inch waists. Other youth-size supporters are One Size, fitting those who measure 20 to 26 inches in the waist. Standard athletic supporters come in Small (26¼ to 32 inches), Medium (32¼ to 38 inches) and Large (38¼ to 44 inches) waist sizes.

The stretchable part of the jockstrap, the part that covers the genitals, is the *same* size from the Small to Large varieties. So if you hear someone bragging about how he had to get a large jockstrap, that doesn't mean he necessarily has a large penis or giant testicles. It means he's simply larger around the waist. (It may also mean that he's an insecure person who feels his personal worth is linked with genital size and/or that he's misinformed or just acting like a jerk!)

Living With Your Growing, Changing Body

As your body grows and changes, there will be times when you feel awkward and embarrassed, times when you wonder if you're normal. You may wonder especially when you get subtle and not-so-subtle messages that bigger is better, that the taller you are or the larger your penis, the more masculine you are. Some of your peers or older relatives may think that "real" men are super-hairy, tough and in control all the time.

In fact, that's not really what being a man means at all. Having a smaller than average penis does *not* make you less of a man, and having a larger than average one does *not* make you more of a man. Neither is lots of chest hair the ultimate measure of masculinity.

While being a man does mean, in part, having your body grow from that of a child to that of an adult, there are many wonderful variations among men. Whether you end up short or tall, slim or stocky, with a little or a lot of body hair—you're still a *normal* man.

It's important to grow to be your *own* man, your own person. This means that you accept the fact that everyone is different in some ways. Some boys develop earlier than others. Some will be shorter or taller than others. Some are naturally more outgoing. Your changes, your physical build and your personal ways of being are all normal—for you. They're all part of what makes you unique. And there's a lot of room in the world for uniqueness!

Being your own man means that you grow to know yourself and what's right for you. It means that you give yourself permission to have feelings—whether they're angry or tender or somewhere in between. You can be gentle and loving as well as assertive and strong. It's a matter of choice, depending on the situation and how you feel. Masculinity is simply gender: It has nothing to do with size or performance or with expressing or holding in certain feelings.

Growing to manhood means learning to like and accept your changing body and the full range of your feelings. What matters most, after all, is the kind of *person* you grow up to be!

5

How Tall Will I Be?

I'm a girl who has such big feet, my dad calls me his "Little Snowshoe Rabbit." But it's NOT funny to me! I'm 4'8" tall and wear a woman's shoe size 7¹/₂! I'm 10 years old and I feel very ugly. ✳ MIMI K.

Can you tell, before you're an adult, about how tall you're going to be? I want to know because I'm 12 and thinking of being a model. But I don't want to ask my parents to pay a lot for modeling lessons and stuff if I'm not going to get tall enough to be a model. I'm 5'2" and I read that models have to be at least 5'7". My mom is only 5'3" and my dad is 5'8", if that makes any difference. ✳ MELODIE G.

How come the girls in my class are mostly taller than the boys (including me)? We had our first junior high dance last weekend and it was sort of embarrassing. There are only two boys in my class who are taller than most of the girls and they danced with everyone. But practically no one, even the shorter girls, wanted to dance with most of us. What upsets me is that I've started to mature in other ways, but I haven't grown very much. I hate to think about always being short and not having any girls like me. ✳ JUSTIN J.

I f you worry about your growing body at times, you're far from alone!

Some young people worry because, like Mimi, they find that their feet grow dramatically before the rest of their body. Growth, in fact, quite often happens in strange (but normal) patterns and, for a time, you may feel awkward with your body. Many young people find that their legs grow before the rest of their body and that their body may grow a lot in height before filling out—with shoulders and chest broadening in boys or hips becoming more rounded in girls.

Others, like Justin, are concerned when they see signs of puberty, but little rapid growth. A girl may find herself towering over her classmates, even the boys, and wonder if it will always be that way . . . or, like Melodie, she may wonder if she will eventually be tall enough to be a model. Lots of boys experience what Justin describes—feeling uncomfortable with being shorter than most of the girls in his class and wondering if he'll ever have a girlfriend.

Everyone has a very individual pattern of growth (see Figs. 5-1 and 5-2). However, it's very common, for a time during junior high, for the girls to be taller than most of the boys. This is because girls tend to start puberty a year or two before boys and reach their peak of growth sometime before the boys in their class do. For most, this is a temporary height imbalance, though some boys will be shorter than average into adulthood and some girls will be taller than average.

The idea that males *must* always be taller than females is a cultural one. Short boys or tall girls can make very good dance partners, dates or friends. Right now you and your classmates may be very self-conscious about height—or lack of it. But luckily such concerns tend to lessen as you get older. There are lots of celebrity couples in which the woman is taller than the man. Your lovability is *not* measured by your height!

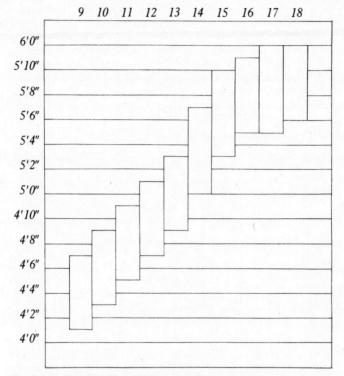

Fig. 5-1 Boys' Height *If you want to compare your height with those of others your age, this chart shows the heights of about 80 percent of boys. Find your age at the top of the chart and your height on the side. The tallest 10 percent and the shortest 10 percent are not on the chart.*

Looking at the top of the bars, you can see that growth levels out for boys at about the age of 17 or 18.

But maybe you just want to know what to expect. How tall are you likely to be as an adult?

Your adult height depends on a number of factors. Young people today tend to be taller than their counterparts of 50 or 100 years ago because nutrition and health care is better these days. But there are some very personal factors that can also influence how tall or short you're likely to be. These include:

■ **Heredity.** Your heredity is a major factor in determining how tall or short you're likely to be. If you have taller than average parents,

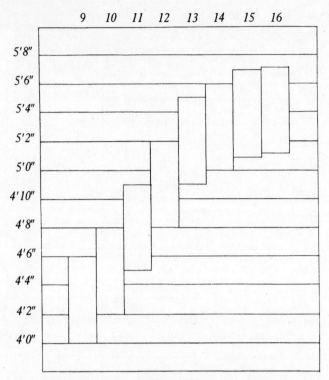

Fig. 5-2 Girls' Height *If you want to see how you measure up to others your age, find your age at the top of the chart and your height on the side. Each bar represents the heights of 80 percent of young people in that age group. The tallest 10 percent and the shortest 10 percent are not on the chart. As you can see, growth levels out for girls at about age 16.*

chances are you, too, will be tall. If both your parents are short, you will probably be fairly short. If one parent is very short and the other taller than average, you may be of medium height or may be closer in stature to one or the other.

If you want to know more specifically what kind of growth to expect, check out the following **"Do the Math! Make a Prediction!"** box.

■ **Stage of development.** If you have few, if any, signs of physical development, delayed puberty may be the cause of your present

Do the Math!
Make a Prediction!

If you're a boy:

1. Add 5 inches to your mother's height: _____

2. Add this sum to your father's height: _____

3. Divide that total sum by 2: _____

Your predicted height: _____

If you're a girl:

1. Subtract 5 inches from your father's height: _____

2. Add this sum to your mother's height: _____

3. Divide that total sum by 2: _____

Your predicted height: _____

short height. Chances are, once puberty begins, you will experience a growth spurt and reach a height that's normal for you. Keep in mind that it's normal for some young people, especially boys, to have some signs of puberty—like genital growth—before really beginning their growth spurt. So if you have a few signs of development and are still shorter than your classmates (and your parents aren't unusually short), you're likely to do quite a lot of growing in the not-too-distant future! For example, a boy who is in stage two of puberty with just the beginning of pubic hair and genital growth can still look forward to a considerable growth spurt—on the average, two or three inches a year for the next three years or so.

However, if you're well into puberty, your growth is likely to be slowing down. As hormone concentration increases in the body, the growth of the long bones—the ones in your legs, for instance—decreases. A girl usually grows to within a half-inch of her maximum height around the time she begins to menstruate. So if you're 12 years old, 5'1" and have already begun to menstruate, your chances of reaching supermodel height requirements are remote.

■ **Special health factors.** There are some special health conditions, such as thyroid problems or chronic kidney disease or rare chromosomal abnormalities such as Turner's syndrome, that can cause unusually short stature. There are other, generally rare, conditions that can cause you to be considerably taller than could be predicted by your heredity. If you are showing signs of unusual height or short stature or if you have any questions about whether you're growing normally, check with your doctor. Help is available!

When Your Height Is A Problem

I'm a boy, 12 years old, and a lot shorter than anyone I know. Is there anything a doctor can do to help me grow taller? ✻ CHRIS H.

There could be many reasons why Chris is a lot shorter than his classmates. A visit to his doctor will help him discover the reason in his case and what, if anything, can or should be done about it.

The doctor will examine him to see how his general health is and whether he has begun puberty. The doctor will also want to know how tall or short his parents are. An x-ray of Chris's hand and wrist—to discover whether bone age matches his chronological age (age in years)—can also give a clue about his growth potential. If, for example, a boy is 12 and the x-ray shows that the bone age of his wrist is 9, that is a sign that there is some retardation of his growth.

In some cases, where a young person shows signs of being significantly shorter than he or she could be genetically, special growth hormones may help. These are used when a preteen or teenager has a medically obvious deficiency of natural growth hormones or is not secreting enough growth hormones from the pituitary gland.

Biosynthetic growth hormones are given by a doctor before puberty actually begins—usually to those who have long been shorter than others their age and whose growth has been slower than usual between the ages of 3 and 12. Recent studies have found that this growth hormone treatment can be given to boys to increase their height and, at the same time, this treatment does not affect their normal timetable of puberty.

It's important to know, however, that these particular hormones are only given to those with proven growth hormone deficiencies and are used only to help those young people reach the height they would have reached without the hormone deficiency. Doctors will not give hormone therapy to those who want to be a lot taller than nature intended. It is not for those who, because of their genetic heritage, are naturally short.

In cases where a normal, healthy boy is between the ages of 14 and 17, is still short and shows no signs of puberty, a doctor may consider treatment with the male hormone testosterone, especially if the boy feels bad about himself and is suffering socially. In a study of a group of such boys at Stanford University, it was shown that those treated for three or four months with testosterone had, by the one-year follow-up, entered puberty and grown up to 4 inches in height. They also felt better about themselves and were much more active in school and social activities than they had been before receiving hormone therapy.

Hormone therapy isn't for everyone, of course. Your doctor may feel that time and growth at your own rate will eventually take care of your particular problem. Or perhaps your body was naturally meant to be shorter than average. But it's worth checking with your doctor anyway to make sure you're normal and to get any medically appropriate help that may be available.

Help! I'm scared that I'm going to be really tall. I'm only 10 years old and am already taller than my mother. And I don't even have any breasts yet. My dad is really tall. I love him a lot, but I don't want to be as tall as he is because I'm a girl and no boys will like me. ✳ TRACY T.

Although Tracy doesn't say just how tall she is now or how tall either of her parents is, it is possible for girls who show signs of being extremely tall—over 6 feet—to have their growth rate slowed and stopped before reaching that height.

It's important to understand, though, that slowing a girl's growth isn't something that should be done on a whim. This treatment usually has to be carefully supervised by a doctor specializing in pediatric endocrinology and is used only for girls meeting certain requirements.

What are these requirements? Usually the girl must be between the ages of 10 and 13 with a medically predicted adult height of more than 6 feet. The doctor also needs to be sure that her present tall stature is not due to any one of a number of rare medical conditions. If she is found to be healthy, normal and unhappy at the thought of becoming so tall, the doctor may consider treating her with the female hormone estrogen to bring on puberty quickly and slow her bone growth.

Hormone therapy to slow growth is much less common for girls today than twenty or even ten years ago. Some feel that it has become much more socially acceptable for women to be tall. Maybe, following the lead of superstar models who *have* to be taller than average to make it in their competitive business, television stars like Lucy Lawless, who gained fame in *Xena, Warrior Princess,* and the rise in the popularity of women's basketball, many girls today feel perfectly fine being taller than average.

It's important to know that some doctors will not use this form of treatment at all, feeling that the risks and side effects of hormone treatment outweigh possible benefits. You and your parents also need to know that there are some side effects to consider. You may experience nausea, excessive weight gain and, perhaps, some menstrual irregularities. And even after treatment, you'll still be fairly tall. If, for example, your final medically predicted height is 6'2", you may, with hormone therapy, be 5'11".

When trying to decide whether hormone therapy is right for you, it's important to think about how much 'difference several inches of height may make in your future life and weigh the benefits against the side effects.

Tall girls and short boys too often feel uncomfortable because our culture tends to expect men to be taller than women. But that doesn't mean you can't be completely healthy, normal and happy even if you're shorter or taller than most people. There are times when it can be an advantage not to be average. Many top athletes are far from average in height. For example, a lot of the best gymnasts—both male and female—are shorter than average. Basketball players are much taller than average. There are some top female models who are close to or well over 6 feet who see their height as a real beauty asset.

Of course, you don't have to be an outstanding athlete or a successful model to feel good about yourself, whatever your height. Taking good care of your body by eating right and keeping active can help you feel healthy and attractive.

Even though you may feel awkward at times while your body is changing and although it may take some time to adjust to being short or tall or in between, there is a lot you can do to feel more comfortable. For example, Chet, 13, who shows signs of being shorter than most of his classmates (he is well into puberty and has one shorter than average parent), has become an avid bodybuilder (many of the top bodybuilders are of less than average height and some of the best power-lifters are short men). He is also learning karate. Chet is strong, healthy, confident—and no one gives him a hard time about being short.

And Megan, who is also 13 and close to 6 feet tall, has started running and taking dance classes to help her feel more at ease with her body and to develop her strength and grace. "Some people tease me, and I don't like that much, but I try to be friendly to everyone," she says. "I think I have a good personality and am making more and more friends. My being tall is something people notice a lot when they don't know me very well, but when they get to know me, other things become more important. And one of these days, when everyone else finishes growing up, I won't be taller than everyone else. I'll always be tall, though. That's part of who I am. And now that I'm getting used to that, I *like* who I am—a lot!"

Getting to know and like yourself—whatever your height—is a vital and wonderful part of growing up!

6

Your Best Weight

How can I keep from getting fat? I'm not fat now, but I don't want to be, because all the kids in my class make fun of this fat girl named Patsy. She doesn't have any friends. I don't want people to hate me like they hate her. Can you tell me how to keep from getting fat or give me a diet that will work for a 9-year-old? ❋ AUDREY B.

I've just been crying my eyes out. I'm 10 and in the fifth grade. It's hard for me because I look much older. I got my period for the first time last year and I'm taller than anyone else in the class. It makes me feel sort of shy. But what was terrible today was that when we were filing out of an assembly, one of the sixth-grade boys who's a monitor thought I wasn't walking fast enough so he said right in front of everyone "Hey, move it, Fats!" I got tears in my eyes right there. My parents say I'm not fat at all, but I don't know whether to believe them. I've been noticing that my hips stick out and I have more fat on my thighs than the other girls in my class. Should I go on a diet? I don't want to be thought of as fat, and I'm scared that all the boys secretly hate me already. ❋ WENDI A.

First off, I admit I'm heavy. I'm 13, 5'5" and weigh more than 200 pounds. But a lot of my friends are heavy, too. It's hard to lose weight, and I've heard that diets aren't any good anyway. But my doctor and my parents are ragging on me about losing weight because I was just diagnosed with diabetes. It's the second type where you take pills instead of getting shots. My doctor says it usually happens in middle-age people but that my weight caused me to get this now. Anyway, everyone is going on about how I need to lose weight and they are clueless about how hard it is! ✲ HUNTER C.

There are two major challenges today in young people maintaining their best, healthiest weight.

One of these is the current national epidemic of obesity among children and teens. The other is *fear* of obesity that drives young people to try diets that can pose a threat to their health and can even result in developing an eating disorder.

The epidemic of obesity is a *new* development that is causing a lot of concern among doctors who treat children and teenagers. Check this out:

- The number of overweight teens has tripled since 1980, and in 1999, some 13 percent of children and teenagers were overweight.

- There are 12 million American children and teens—22 percent of this young generation—who are significantly overweight.

- Although the obesity epidemic cuts across all ethnic groups, those who are at greatest risk are African American and Latino teens and those of all ethnicities who are growing up in families who are in poverty or living on very limited budgets.

■ The increase in adolescent obesity has led to a major increase in the number of teens being diagnosed with adult type (Type II) diabetes, before now rarely seen in anyone under the age of 40. Diabetes is a serious disease that also puts you at risk for some life-threatening and life-changing health problems, such as heart disease and blindness.

■ In January 2002, the U.S. Surgeon General declared childhood and adolescent obesity a national epidemic!

Why is all this happening??
There are several reasons that teens today are more likely to be fat. Think about it. Do any of these make sense for you—or your friends?

■ More schools are dropping the physical education requirements, so young people are getting less and less exercise at school. In the past, would-be couch potatoes at least had to move around a little in PE class if nowhere else. Less exercise = more fat.

■ Because of concerns about traffic, distance, weather and crime, fewer parents today are comfortable letting their kids walk to school or to other activities. So young people today are less active in yet another way than those ten or twenty years ago.

■ School cafeterias have changed. Now more and more are selling fast foods, junk foods and sodas. Even if you don't have a brand-name fast-food franchise on campus, does your cafeteria offer things like cheeseburgers, nachos and chicken nuggets? Enough said! Years ago, school cuisine might have been totally lame but tended to do less damage weight-wise.

■ High tech—rather than sports or other physical activities—is #1 in after school activities. What do *you* do after school? If you're like many young preteens or teens, you probably come home, get in front of the computer and play games or surf the Internet or watch TV. It's tough to burn the calories of those after-school snacks when you're sitting still!

How do you know if you're too fat?

You can't always tell by looking in the mirror. For example, Wendi's classmates might think she's fat, but the fact is that Wendi is an "early bloomer" who is going through her physical development early. A certain amount of weight gain is a natural part of that process. As a more physically mature female than her classmates are at the moment, it's normal for Wendi to have wider hips and more fat padding on her body. At the peak of her growth spurt, the average girl will grow about 3½ inches and gain close to 20 pounds in one year! That change can feel pretty huge. But it doesn't mean a person is fat. She just has a more grown-up shape.

There are other factors in trying to figure out if you're truly over-weight—or not!

One of these factors is body type. The three most common body types (see Figs. 6-1 to 6-3) are *ectomorphs,* who tend to be naturally thin and angular in build; *endomorphs,* who tend to be rounder, have more body fat and softer curves; and *mesomorphs,* who are muscular, with broad shoulders and slim hips.

So if you're basically an endomorph, you may be at your ideal weight yet look heavier than an ectomorph friend of the same weight. Some of the models and actresses you admire, besides being under-weight, may also have a more angular body type than yours. If that happens to be the case, you can never really look like they do, no mat-ter how much weight you try to lose!

Genes are important in determining your body shape and size. If you have parents who are significantly overweight, you may need to be especially careful about what you eat and exercise regularly in order to avoid obesity. Studies of people who were adopted as children have

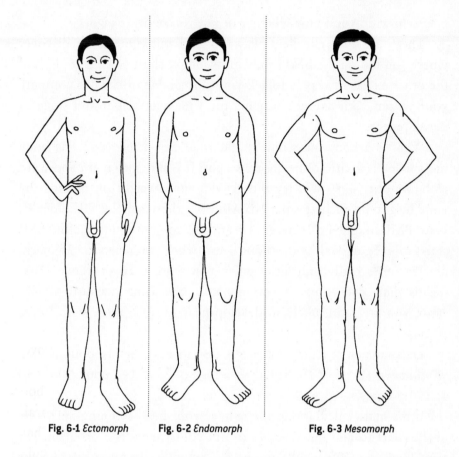

Fig. 6-1 *Ectomorph*   **Fig. 6-2** *Endomorph*   **Fig. 6-3** *Mesomorph*

found that their weight and body shape more closely matches those of their biological parents rather than their adoptive parents. Also, certain ethnic groups are more likely to have a higher percentage of overweight people. This may be due to a combination of genetics, shared eating habits and cultural preferences (not all cultures are hung up on thinness as a necessity for beauty). In a study of overweight children and teens by ethnicity, the Centers for Disease Control found that 11.6 percent of white males and 9.6 percent of white females were overweight, while 12.5 percent of African American males and 16.3 percent of African American females were overweight. Among Latino children and teens, 15 percent of males and 14 percent of females were overweight.

So how do you know whether or not you're overweight?

There are two excellent ways to find out: One is to discover where you fall on the BMI (body mass index) chart (see Fig. 6-4), and the other excellent way is to ask your doctor. He or she can compare your weight with average weights for your age, height and stage of development.

What is a body mass index, and what can it tell you? The body mass index is a ratio of height to weight. If you're into math and want to figure out your own, try this: Divide your weight (in pounds) by your height (in inches) squared. Multiply the result by 705. Ideally, your BMI should be between 19 and 22 for optimum health. BMI starts looking unhealthy (for your heart) when you reach the 25 mark, and becomes really unhealthy when you score a 26 or above. That means that, over time, if you maintain the same height-to-weight ratio, you are more likely to develop heart disease those with lower BMIs.

Let's say you're a girl who is 5'4" (64 inches). At 116 pounds, you would have a BMI of 20. You'd hit a BMI of 25 at 145 pounds and 30 at 174 pounds.

If the math calculations above have your head spinning, just look at the chart to find out whether or not your weight is a problem. Put your finger on your height and go across until you reach the number closest to your weight. Then trace straight down to reach the bottom number in bold type. *That* is your BMI.

Help! I'm Too Skinny!

I have a problem with being too skinny. I'm 14, in middle school and no girls will go out with me because I'm not what they call a hunk. Is there something I could eat or do or medicine to take to change my body fast? ✻ MARK K.

Fat or Fit?
Finding Your BMI (Body Mass Index)

Height	Body Weight												
4'10"	91	96	100	105	110	115	119	124	129	134	138	143	148
4'11"	94	99	104	109	114	119	124	128	133	138	143	148	153
5'0"	97	102	107	112	118	123	128	133	138	143	148	153	158
5'1"	100	106	111	116	122	127	132	137	143	148	153	158	164
5'2"	104	109	115	120	126	131	136	142	147	153	158	164	169
5'3"	107	113	118	124	130	135	141	146	152	158	163	169	175
5'4"	110	116	122	128	134	140	145	151	157	163	169	174	180
5'5"	114	120	126	132	138	144	150	156	162	168	174	180	186
5'6"	118	124	130	136	142	148	155	161	167	173	179	186	192
5'7"	121	127	134	140	146	153	159	166	172	178	185	191	197
5'8"	125	131	138	144	151	158	164	171	177	184	190	197	203
5'9"	128	135	142	149	155	162	169	176	182	189	196	203	209
5'10"	132	139	146	153	160	167	174	181	188	195	202	207	215
5'11"	136	143	150	157	165	172	179	186	193	200	208	215	222
6'0"	140	147	154	162	169	177	184	191	199	206	213	221	228
BMI	19	20	21	22	23	24	25	26	27	28	29	30	31

Fig. 6-4

Feeling embarrassed by a skinny body can be as painful as worrying about fat, as incredible as that may seem to those who say they can gain weight just by *looking* at food!

If you, like Mark, are worried about being skinny, you need to first check with your doctor to make sure that all is well. If your doctor says you're healthy but on the low end of your weight range or even a bit below that, here are some things to think about.

■ *This may be a temporary way of being.* You may be in the middle of your big growth spurt, and that takes a lot of calories. As your growth rate slows down, you may start to fill out.

■ *You may be just naturally slender.* Remember the body types we saw earlier in this chapter? You may have a naturally lean, angular (ectomorphic) body type. Even so, with good nutrition and an active exercise program, you may build a strong, though slender, body. Also, you can dress in ways that make you look attractively or athletically slender instead of skinny. As time goes on, and your body burns fewer calories, you may find your weight increasing a little.

■ *Make exercise part of your daily routine.* Regular exercise that includes weight training can help you to build a healthy, strong body with greater muscle definition. Working out with weights can give a lean body more curves, whether you're male or female, and help you look and feel stronger.

■ *Change eating behavior that keeps you too skinny.* Keep a diary of everything you eat for at least a week and notice your habits. Are you skipping meals a lot? When you're upset, do you stop eating? Do you forget to eat or simply don't have time? Note how much or how little you actually eat. This can give you some important clues for change. Never skip a meal. Even when you're upset, try to eat regular meals. Your body needs essential nutrients no matter what you're feeling!

■ *Don't try to gain weight with unhealthy food.* There are better ways. Don't snack on candy and other junk foods. Treat your body to snacks such as granola, bread and peanut butter, fruits and vegetables. The same foods, in greater quantity, that can help your overweight friends lose weight can also give *you* the healthy body you want.

■ *RUN from quick fixes!* There's no substitute for building your body the healthy, sane way: by eating healthy foods and following a regular exercise program. Some young men hope to build impressive physiques by taking anabolic steroids—and that's a BIG mistake!! Unfortunately, a lot of young teens, both male and female, are taking steroids to look good—and end up getting a lot more than just a big disappointment. See the special bulletin below.

Warning: Steroids Are Hazardous to
Your Health and Your Looks!

Many young people, wanting to look muscular and athletic, take anabolic steroids. A survey funded by the National Institute on Drug Abuse found that nearly as many middle school students as high school students were taking these dangerous substances.

What exactly *are* anabolic steroids? These are hormones, often variations of the male hormone testosterone, that can be taken in pill or injection form. Some teens combine these with stimulants or painkillers (this is called "stacking") or taking varying doses—increasing then decreasing doses, a practice called "pyramiding."

What are the dangers of steroids?

1. If you inject steroids and share needles (or use ones not properly sterilized), you may be at risk for HIV or hepatitis infection.

2. Your growth may be terminated prematurely if you take steroids during your growth spurt—and you'll end up shorter than you would have been otherwise.

3. Boys can also suffer acne, a reduction in the size of their testicles, impotence, baldness and irreversible breast enlargement. Who needs all that?

4. Girls can end up with acne, deep voices, loss of hair on the head and more body hair, including facial and chest hair—not exactly great for your body image!

5. Both sexes risk life-threatening side effects like high blood pressure and blood clotting, which can increase risks for heart attacks or strokes (at young ages!) and potentially fatal liver cysts.

6. You can have some unpleasant personality changes not likely to add to your popularity or your general quality of life: aggression, fighting and other violent behavior.

REMEMBER:
Quick fixes like steroids = trouble!
Build your strong body the slow, sane way:
by eating well and exercising sensibly.

Help! I'm Afraid Of Getting Fat!

A lot of the girls I know both at school and in ballet class are dieting and I'm afraid if I don't I'll get fat, but my mom won't let me. She is always going on about me having a balanced diet and says there's no need for dieting and it's unhealthy. I'm scared that I'll get fat and everyone will hate me and I'll get kicked out of ballet class (we get weighed every week). Help! ✳ JILLIANE J.

Many young people like Jilliane are under a lot of pressure to stay slender and are afraid of getting fat for a lot of reasons. If all the people you know are dieting and almost competing with each other to eat less and be the skinniest person around, you may fear losing all your friends if you gain even a tiny amount of weight. If you're involved in a sport like figure skating or gymnastics or, for guys, wrestling, where maintaining a slender body shape is important, you may feel intense pressure to diet. The same is true if dancing, especially ballet, happens to be your passion.

You're also more at risk for an eating disorder if:

■ You're a teen (or almost a teen) and very conscious of being judged by how you look.

■ You're a perfectionist: You're probably a good student and well behaved if you're at risk for or are actually developing anorexia. Those with bulimia are a bit more rebellious.

■ Weight is important in your family—either one or both of your parents puts a lot of importance on being slim.

■ You have some history of trauma or abuse, often sexual, and feel safer with a body that's not outstanding or attention-getting.

■ You're an early bloomer. Especially girls who reach puberty early may have poor body image.

What kind of eating disorders are there?

FEAR OF OBESITY SYNDROME

What is it? This can be an early warning of more serious eating disorders, like anorexia nervosa, because it involves an exaggerated fear of fat and self-induced malnutrition. It isn't as intense as anorexia, but some of the behavior is the same.

Symptoms: Teens with Fear of Obesity Syndrome avoid food as much as possible, diet very strictly and worry about being fat when they're really not.

Why it's dangerous: Fear of Obesity Syndrome can evolve into anorexia nervosa or bulimia. It can also interfere with your growth and development because you're not getting the nutrition your body needs at this special time in your life. As we saw in the previous chapters, your body needs nutrients and a certain level of body fat to complete the growth and maturation process. And besides, if your body shape isn't supermodel angular, no amount of dieting and deprivation is going to make you look like your favorite model or actress.

If this might be a problem for you: Talk with your parents and your physician. You can get nutritional and behavioral counseling to help you develop an eating and exercise plan that's healthy for you.

ANOREXIA NERVOSA

What is it? This is a serious physical and emotional disorder that causes people, usually girls but sometimes boys as well, to diet and exercise compulsively, losing so much weight that they become dangerously thin. Studies have suggested that anorexia nervosa is a complex disorder that may have physical, hormonal, as well as emotional causes.

Symptoms: People with anorexia avoid food (except they may be obsessed with cooking it for others while not eating it themselves), exercise compulsively, may use laxatives heavily and make themselves vomit if they do slip and eat something they feel they shouldn't. Those who have had this disorder for a while experience dangerous weight loss, sometimes looking like living skeletons, even as they insist they could still lose more weight.

Why it's dangerous: Five to fifteen percent of those with anorexia nervosa actually die of this disorder. But those who survive may still suffer from severe malnutrition, very low blood pressure, irregular heartbeat, bone weakness and general poor health.

If this might be a problem for you: Those who love you are probably already voicing a lot of concern. It's very important to get medical help right away. Sometimes you can get help from a medical team that will help you to deal with the emotional as well as physical aspects of this disorder. If your symptoms are especially severe, you may need to be hospitalized for a while until any life-threatening complications can be treated. Even though you may feel you don't really have a problem, listen to the concern of others and see a doctor today! Your future health—even your life—could depend on it.

BULIMIA

What is it? Bulimia is also a disorder that has both physical and emotional characteristics. People with bulimia are usually within their normal weight range but go on eating binges, where they will eat a lot of food and then, to avoid gaining weight, will use vomiting and laxatives to purge the food from their systems. Many people with bulimia have also been found to suffer from depression.

Symptoms: Because a lot of the behavior of bulimia is secretive and because there may be no dramatic weight loss to show that something is wrong, people with bulimia can go on for years without anyone discovering their problem. However, some symptoms like severe tooth decay (because of stomach acids eating away tooth enamel during frequent bouts of vomiting), irritated mouth tissues and swollen salivary glands are common symptoms.

Why it's dangerous: Bulimia can also destroy your health and even kill you. In addition to possible ulcers, hernia and kidney and heart failure due to dangerous body chemistry imbalances, those with bulimia can also die as a result of a ruptured esophagus from vomiting or from ipecac poisoning (some people with bulimia take this daily to induce vomiting) or a heart attack.

If this might be a problem for you: Tell your parents or another adult who loves you and get immediate medical care. Treatment is usually a combination of medication (to treat depression) as well as psychotherapy.

COMPULSIVE OVEREATING

What is it? People with this eating disorder eat a lot, often because of feelings they're having—from sadness to anger to plain boredom—rather than from hunger. Because those with this disorder don't make themselves throw up, they tend to range from somewhat overweight to dangerously obese (more than 20 percent over their ideal weight).

Symptoms: Eating large quantities of food, often in secret. Compulsive overeaters will often eat normally at mealtimes but then binge when they're alone. Food is often used to relieve stress or to push down angry feelings that the person can't express in words.

Type II Diabetes Alert

This used to be a disease of middle age and was never seen in children or teenagers. But now, with so many young people suffering from obesity, a rising number of teens are being diagnosed with Type II (also called adult-onset) diabetes.

See your doctor right away if:

■ You weigh more than 20 percent over your ideal weight. You may have Type II diabetes without realizing it.

■ You have noticed that you're unusually thirsty and/or have been urinating a lot more often.

■ You've noticed a thick, velvety pigmentation of the skin, especially around your neck and elbows.

Untreated diabetes can lead to kidney failure, high blood pressure, blindness and other serious health problems.

Why it's dangerous: Being significantly overweight or obese is not only hazardous to your social life and good feelings about yourself, but is also dangerous to your health. It is estimated that 80 percent of obese teenagers go on to become obese adults. And obesity is a major risk factor for Type II diabetes, heart disease and some forms of cancer.

If this might be a problem for you: Consult your physician for referral to a supervised nutritional program such as Shapedown. Sometimes individual or family therapy can also help treat some of the painful feelings that may be a big part of this disorder.

Help! My Weight Is A Definite Problem!

My doctor says I have to lose about 10 pounds, but he didn't say anything about a diet and my mom is on this total diet tear. I can't find anything decent to eat. Just cottage cheese, fruit, vegetables I hate and so much popcorn I don't care if I never see it again! I heard that dieting isn't good for people my age (13). How can I convince my mom? ✻ MARK Y.

What diet is best if you have to lose a lot of weight? I'm supposed to lose a lot of weight, like about 50 pounds, and I keep hearing different things—like dieting is totally bad, or one diet is good but all the others are bad and that some foods help you lose weight. Could you tell me what to do because I'm going to be having to lose weight for a long time and I don't want to be totally bored—or worse, having to eat everything I hate and nothing I like. Help! ✻ SAMANTHA C.

Dieting in the traditional sense—carrot sticks, cottage cheese and severely restricted calories—isn't a good idea for anyone, but especially young people who are in their prime growing years. This time of your life is not a good time to try unhealthy fad diets that deprive you of essential nutrients. What harm can dieting do?

Dieting can stunt your growth. During this time of growth and change, you need plenty of vitamins, minerals and other nutrients to help bone growth. If you cut back severely in calories at this point in your life, you could permanently stunt your growth.

For example, in a recent New York study, doctors found that 14 adolescents between the ages of 9 and 17 who had been on strict, self-imposed diets were not only underweight for their ages, but were also underdeveloped and shorter than they should have been. All said that they skipped meals or ate small portions because they were afraid of getting fat. When they began to eat normally again, some of the younger children started to grow again. However, several of the older adolescents studied had permanently stunted bones. Another interesting finding: None of the fourteen got fat when they ate normally.

Dieting can interfere with physical development. If you don't get adequate nutrition and are seriously underweight, your puberty may be delayed.

In studies of young female ballet dancers in New York, Dr. Jeanne Brooks-Gunn compared the weights and menstrual histories of three groups of young women all about the same height: 5'4". The non-dancers studied weighed, on the average, 125 pounds. The first group of dancers weighed an average of 115. Both of these groups had similar development patterns, with the average girl beginning to menstruate at about 12 or 13 and, in time, establishing a regular pattern of periods. In the third and lowest-weight group of dancers, those weighing an average of 105 pounds, however, puberty was delayed. Dr. Brooks-Gunn has observed that the dancers, especially the lightest ones, tend to maintain their low weight via strict dieting.

You need a certain amount of body fat—for females, it's between 17 and 22 percent of total body weight—to stimulate hormones that trigger and regulate menstrual periods. If you fall below this critical balance, you may begin to skip menstrual periods or stop menstruating altogether.

Doctors don't yet know for sure what, if anything, happens to your body if you don't menstruate regularly, but some believe that low body fat can cause lowered hormone levels and, quite possibly, the loss of calcium, resulting in bone weakness.

Whether you want to lose weight, gain weight or just maintain your present weight, it makes sense to eat regular, balanced, healthy meals. Being smart about your eating can help you stay healthy and weigh what you should.

How do you get smart and start eating right? First, you need to learn about the foods your body needs to be healthy and active and look terrific. You need to know how to mix the foods your body needs with the occasional treats you really want. Second, you can learn how to get active and build a strong, trim, great-looking body. Commonsense eating and exercise work together, making it easier for you, as you begin to feel and look better, to do what's best for you and your growing body.

EATING FOR GOOD HEALTH

Eating for good health means eating reasonable amounts of a lot of different foods (see Fig. 6-5). Getting a good balance of nutrients helps you feel better and look better. For best results, choose foods from the four basic food groups every day:

MEAT AND OTHER PROTEIN-RICH FOODS

(three 2-ounce servings daily)

This category includes not only meat such as beef, pork, lamb, chicken or turkey, but also fish, seafood, eggs, peanut butter and tofu.

FRUITS AND VEGETABLES

(four or more servings daily; one serving = 1 piece fresh fruit, ½ cup cooked fruit or vegetable)

This category of foods can bring you a variety of essential vitamins and leave you feeling full without adding too many extra calories to your diet. Get into the habit, at least part of the time, of substituting

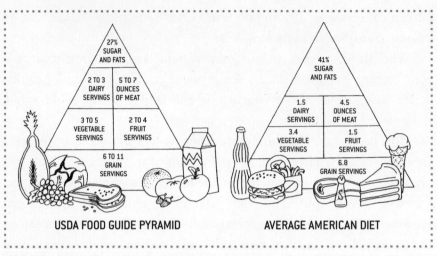

USDA FOOD GUIDE PYRAMID   AVERAGE AMERICAN DIET

Fig. 6-5 *The Pyramid on the left shows the ideal American diet, while the Pyramid on the right shows the average American diet—with way too much sugar and fat.*

fruit for sugary snacks. Fresh peaches, strawberries, apples, oranges, pears, bananas, watermelon and kiwi fruit—just to name a few possibilities—can make wonderful, satisfying sweet snacks. And vegetables such as green beans, broccoli, mushrooms, lettuce, cauliflower and celery can add a lot to any meal.

BREADS, PASTA, CEREAL AND STARCHY VEGETABLES

(four or more servings daily; one serving = 1 slice of bread or ½ cup cooked pasta, starchy vegetables or cereal)

This food category is a must for everyone—even those who are watching their weight. To maintain energy levels, you need carbohydrates, which is what this category includes. Just watch what you put on them, as well as the amounts you eat. In this category are things like bread, pasta, rice, beans, carrots, peas, onions, potatoes and corn. It's best if you can eat these carbohydrates closer to their natural state than those that have been super-processed. For example, whole wheat bread, preferably stone ground, is better for you than white bread, and brown rice is a better food choice than white rice. In the same way, corn, on the cob or not, will give you more nutrients and far fewer calories than a corn muffin.

MILK AND MILK PRODUCTS

(two to three 1-cup servings daily)

This group doesn't just include milk of all kinds, but also yogurt, ice cream and ice milk.

Commonsense eating means balance in this as well as every other category. Three cups of ice cream a day doesn't make good nutritional sense, especially if you're overweight. Try a *variety* of milk products, including low-fat yogurt and low-fat soft and hard cheese. You may find some new food favorites!

Just to make sure you're getting the proper vitamins, it's a good idea—in addition to eating a balanced diet—to take a multivitamin tablet daily, preferably one containing iron as well.

> *I have this problem: I hate almost everything that's good for me. Vegetables of all kinds make me want to throw up. Yogurt is totally disgusting and so is skim milk. How can I eat healthy stuff when I hate everything except hamburgers, potato chips, ice cream and chocolate pudding?* ✳ CINDY D.

Even if you're a picky eater, you can build a balanced daily eating plan based on the four basic food groups. Some of these are ideas you can try yourself. Some are ones you might talk over with whoever does most of the cooking at your house.

IF YOU HATE VEGETABLES

Approach them in a new way. If you've learned to hate them cooked, eat them raw as often as possible. If you can't face canned vegetables, try some fresh or frozen varieties.

Some confirmed vegetable-haters, for example, find that eating sliced raw vegetables such as carrots, celery, green pepper rings, cauliflower and broccoli with a low-fat cottage cheese or yogurt dip is much easier and more fun than facing a plate full of cooked vegetables.

You can sneak new vegetable varieties into your meals by eating just a little mixed in with vegetables you can tolerate better. For example, maybe you wouldn't dream of eating cauliflower by itself, but if it's mixed with corn, broccoli and red peppers, you may find that it's really okay. (There are some frozen vegetable medleys like the above that come already mixed to make it easier for you or your parents to prepare.)

New seasonings, some lemon juice, a spoonful of grated Parmesan cheese or a bit of cheese sauce can help give new taste sensations to vegetables that you may even find you like after all!

YOU HATE MILK

Try the milk products *least* disgusting to you. If you're not too sure about yogurt, try frozen yogurt first. Or mix regular low-fat yogurt with fruit. Get some of your milk allotment with cereal, puddings and custards. Make yourself a blender shake using skim or low-fat milk and fruit you especially like.

IF YOU DON'T LIKE MEAT

Concentrate on other protein sources such as eggs, cheese, peanut butter and tofu, which has long been used in Asian foods and is now more and more popular as a meat substitute in everything from chili to lasagna.

If your family insists that you eat meat, very small pieces, cut up and mixed with rice and vegetables, may be easier to take.

IF YOU HATE FISH

Try some different varieties. Some fish tastes very "fishy" and some doesn't. If you don't like bland fish, try putting extra spices, seasonings or lemon juice on your portion. You could be pleasantly surprised!

Help For Eating Problems

IF YOU LIKE TO SNACK A LOT

Start snacking on food that's good for you. Cut out or cut down on cookies, candy, brownies, pastries and salty chips. Instead, try raw vegetables, nuts, raisins, fruit and low-fat cheeses.

IF YOU CRAVE SWEETS

Eat fruit as often as this craving strikes. If you must have sugar, limit the amounts. Try one scoop of ice cream instead of two or angel food cake instead of frosted layer cake.

IF YOU AND YOUR FRIENDS LIKE FAST FOODS

Although hamburgers or tacos or pizza may be okay as an occasional treat, these fast foods shouldn't be a part of your daily eating habits. These all contain nutrients your body can use. But these fast foods shouldn't make up your whole diet. Particularly if you are overweight, watch your portions and try to make them a special treat rather than an everyday meal choice.

It's also possible to go to a fast-food restaurant these days and *not* eat lots of fatty, high-calorie foods. More and more places are offering salad bars, baked potatoes and vegetables. So you can have just as much fun with your friends and be good to your body, too!

IF YOU'RE A BREAKFAST SKIPPER

Don't! No matter how unappetizing breakfast may seen, eat something. If you're in a rush, take along a carton of low-fat or fat-free yogurt and a piece of fruit. If you can make time for a sit-down breakfast, a bowl of oatmeal with a little brown sugar mixed with your favorite fruit will keep you from getting too hungry (and eating everything you can get your hands on) later. A lot of teens (and older people, too) who have weight problems skip breakfast and sometimes even lunch. Then they fill the evening with a big dinner (because by that time, they're *really* starving!) and high-calorie snacks.

IF YOU EAT WHEN YOU'RE UPSET . . . OR BORED

If you're looking to relieve anger and tension, don't load up on bread or sweets! Head out for a vigorous walk and get some of that steam out of your system. Write in your diary. Talk your feelings over with a friend. All of the above will help you feel a lot better afterward, while overeating can just make you feel worse.

If you head for comfort food—sweets, potato chips, macaroni and cheese (those instant microwaveable packets are just *too* convenient as snacks after a particularly bad day at school) or fast foods—when you're upset, make a list of healthy and pleasurable activities to soothe your feelings. Talk your problem over with someone who cares. Or get active: Walk, run, swim or even just hit a tennis ball as hard as you can against a sturdy outside wall.

IF YOU ARE AFRAID YOU WON'T LOSE WEIGHT UNLESS YOU GO ON A STRICT DIET

Look at it this way: How long have you ever been able to stay on a very restrictive diet? It is much better to make slight, healthy changes to your lifestyle and eating habits. That way, you'll be able to stick to these changes instead of being on the "feast or famine" treadmill—

dieting strictly and then, in total boredom or desperation, eating everything you've felt deprived of, then dieting again. This isn't a race to try
to lose 10 pounds overnight. That can't be done in a healthy way, and
bizarre, fad diets don't lead to lasting weight loss.

A better way to reach or maintain a healthy weight: Take your
time. Make little but important changes to your daily meals and
snacks. Get active. Discover new interests and hobbies that can fight
the boredom that drives you to the cookie jar. You'll be amazed how
much easier this is than dieting and how much better you'll feel!

IF YOU'RE REALLY OVERWEIGHT

Check with your physician before beginning any weight loss program.
Girls in their teens typically need about 2,000 to 2,400 calories a day,
and adolescent boys need about 2,700 calories daily to maintain their
current weights. Cutting down even a few hundred calories a day—
either by eliminating a snack or exercising regularly—can help you
lose weight slowly. During these important growth years, you should
never eat fewer than 1,200 calories a day—and it's best to get your
doctor's advice before you even cut down that much.

Some young people find organizations such as Weight Watchers
helpful. Some chapters of Weight Watchers even have special meetings
just for teens. There are also special summer camp programs spon-
sored by Weight Watchers and other weight loss groups. If you prefer
to lose weight on your own, you must be careful to get proper nutrition, so do consult your doctor before trying to lose weight. He or she
can help you decide how much weight you need to lose and the best
way to do it.

Your doctor will also probably tell you that the best way for you to
lose weight if you need to is not by dieting but by exercise. It's true!
Eating tends to be less of a problem for overweight preteens and teens
than inactivity. Many overweight young people don't eat any more—
and may actually eat less—than their slim classmates. But studies show
that they exercise a lot less.

Food Habits That Are Hazardous to Your Health

Food Hazards	How These Are Hazardous	Foods to Avoid or Cut Back	Good Food Substitutes
Soft drinks/ Caffeine	1. Can add to stomach acidity 2. Can add empty calories 3. Can contribute to sleep disorders and heart rhythm disturbances	Sugary soft drinks Colas (no more than two a day **at most!**) Coffee Bottled iced tea with sugar	WATER is #1! (Drink at least eight glasses a day!) Fruit juice Vegetable juice Herbal tea Green tea
Sugar	1. A factor in obesity, heart disease, diabetes and hypoglycemia 2. Contributes to tooth decay 3. Personality and behavior problems	Sugary soft drinks Candy, cake, cookies Ice cream Convenience foods (packaged meals or fast food may have lots of sugar)	Fruit Fresh foods you prepare or get from a restaurant salad bar
Salt	1. Can be factor in high blood pressure 2. Can increase PMS water retention	Canned soups and vegetables Frozen convenience foods Snacks like potato and corn chips Fast food (even milkshakes have high salt content)	Lemon juice or herbal seasonings as salt substitute Fresh meals you make yourself or soups and frozen entrées that are low-sodium (check labels!)
Fat	Contributes to obesity, heart disease (which can start in adolescence!) and certain cancers	Fried foods Bacon, sausage and spareribs Butter, margarine, fatty dressings Snacks like like donuts, chips or rich nuts (like macadamia nuts)	Lean meats and fish that are baked or broiled Low-fat or nonfat dairy products (including low-fat yogurt or nonfat sour cream as a potato topping) Low-fat or nonfat salad dressings

Good Food on the Run
**YES! It's possible to enjoy fast food with your friends
if you make good substitutions!**

INSTEAD OF . . .	TRY THIS!
High-fat burgers and sandwiches or potato salad, French fries or onion rings	Salad bars (greens, fruit, veggies—no creamy salads—e.g., potato, macaroni or ambrosia) with low-fat, nonfat or minimum amount of dressing
Cheeseburger	Hamburger
Fried chicken, fish sandwich or chicken nuggets	Chicken breast sandwich or chicken fajita pita
Fried fish sticks	Seafood salad
Fried tacos and burritos	Soft tacos and burritos
Meat pizza	Vegetarian pizza
Milkshake	Plain or chocolate low-fat or nonfat milk
Cola	Water with lemon slices or iced tea (with no sugar)

If your favorite pastimes are watching TV, reading and going to the movies—you can still do what you enjoy, but you also need to squeeze in some *active* pursuits as well. A study from Harvard and the New England Medical Center showed that TV watching can make you fat! The doctors studied more than 13,000 kids between the ages of 6 and 17 over a period of years. Those who watched the most TV were also the most likely to be overweight in childhood and/or to become obese in adolescence.

Things like watching TV and going to the movies can be especially fattening because not only are you sitting and inactive, but you are also often eating high-calorie snacks at the same time. Getting your excess weight off can begin with not eating while watching TV or

The Top Ten
Most Nutritious Vegetables
How many do you like?
Which ones do you think you could learn to like?

1. Broccoli

2. Spinach

3. Brussels sprouts

4. Lima beans

5. Peas

6. Asparagus

7. Artichokes

8. Cauliflower

9. Sweet potatoes

10. Carrots

Hungry?
These Foods Are Tops In Satisfying Hunger!

1. Potatoes (baked, not French fries!)

2. Fish (broiled or grilled, not fried!)

3. Oatmeal

4. Oranges

5. Apples

6. Whole-wheat pasta

7. Beef steak (preferably lean)

8. Grapes

9. Air-popped popcorn

10. Bran cereal

Guidelines for Healthy Weight Loss

(Courtesy of Dept. of Nutritional Services,
Kaiser Permanente Medical Group, San Francisco)

Food Group	Daily Serving	One Serving Examples
Protein	2	2 eggs 2–3 oz. poultry, fish, meat 3–4 oz. tuna 1 cup beans/lentils 4 Tbsp. peanut butter
Milk products	4	1 cup yogurt 2 cups cottage cheese 1 cup milk 2 slices cheese
Breads and starches	4	½ cup hot cereal ¾ cup dry cereal 1 slice bread 1 tortilla ½ hamburger bun ½ cup rice, noodles, pasta
Fruits and vegetables	4	1 whole fruit ½ cup fruit juice 1 cup vegetables

reading or are at the movies or anyplace except at regular meals. You'll also look better and feel better when you stop sitting and start moving!

Get Active For Good Health!

Exercise is vital for good health and good looks! Regular aerobic exercise—that means exercise vigorous enough to give your whole body a workout and increase your heart rate—helps keep body organs such as your heart and lungs working well and also strengthens your bones. Regular exercise—more than anything else at this time in your life—

can help you keep your weight where you want it and gives you more energy and stamina.

Regular exercise can also be good for your feelings. Studies have shown that keeping active helps you overcome stress, anxiety, depression and general moodiness.

For best results, you need to do some sort of vigorous exercise at least three times a week. It's easier to stick to this if you find a type of exercise you like or can at least tolerate.

Some of the best forms of exercise include: brisk walking, running, swimming, jumping rope, bicycling (regular or on a stationary cycle), dancing (aerobic, ballet, tap, jazz), cross-country skiing, vigorous racquetball, vigorous ice skating or roller-skating.

The right exercise for you depends not only on your personal tastes, but also on your circumstances right now.

■ **If you're out of shape and/or very overweight:** Ease into an exercise program. Try regular walking or lap swimming. Or get on your bicycle. If you're embarrassed that others will see you, try an indoor stationary cycle or exercise to videotape exercise programs (try the low-impact aerobic varieties).

■ **If you tend to get bored and quit exercising again and again:** Commit yourself in a new way. Sign up for a class at your local Y or Girls or Boys Club or make a pact with a friend or family member for regular exercise sessions. Taking an evening walk with your mom or dad, for example, can be a good way for you both to get in shape and have time together for private talks or just to enjoy each other's company.

■ **If you burn out on exercise or get hurt easily:** Pick a sport that's low risk and tolerable. Start exercising slowly and gradually build up your strength. If you've been inactive and then try to run 5 miles, of course you'll have aches and pains and decide the pain isn't worth it. Take time to warm up before you exercise, and wear the proper exercise attire.

■ Seek advice from your parents, your gym teacher or sports-minded friends or relatives in choosing exercise shoes or equipment. Proper shoes are especially important for sports such as running, aerobic dance and fast walking.

Don't overdo your physical fitness efforts. Working out at a new and vigorous sport more than four times a week can hurt your body. You need to let your muscles rest for about 48 hours between workouts to heal.

With the proper rest, warm-up and exercise equipment and attire, you're less likely to be injured, discouraged, bored or burned out. You'll also be more likely to stick to and really enjoy your active new life!

When you think about it, it really doesn't have to take that much time or effort to eat and exercise for good health. But what a difference it all can make in the way you feel about yourself!

7

Caring for Your Changing Body

My mom nags me all the time to take a bath. She has always done this, but it's getting worse now that I'm almost 12. Why should I have to take more baths now just because I'm older? ✳ BRAD K.

I'm the only person in my school who sweats. Honest! My hands sweat all the time. My underarms sweat constantly. Even my feet sweat! I feel horrible about it and scared that people will notice and make fun of me. What can I do? ✳ LESLEY G.

Everyone else I know at school looks really cool. But I can't pull things together. My hair is awful. I'm starting to get zits on my face. My nails are a disaster area! How can I look prettier and more like my friends? ✳ ASHLEY J.

Caring for your changing body means learning new grooming skills and unlearning some old kids' tactics.

What are some old tactics that won't work for you anymore now that you're growing up?

Fake baths. Splashing water on your hands or face or feet (or wherever else your parents are likely to check or notice) and pretending that you took a bath or shower.

Underwear marathons. Seeing how long you can wear one pair of underwear before your mother notices.

The Toothbrush Tease. Wetting your toothbrush to make people think you brushed your teeth—when you really didn't.

The After-Gym Sprint. Dashing out of gym class ahead of everyone else to avoid taking a shower.

Why won't kids' tactics work for you anymore? Because you're not a little kid! Now that you're growing up, your changing body needs new and different care.

Your sweat glands are becoming more active. This means you perspire more in general, but underarm perspiration may be the most noticeable to you. Sometimes it may seem as if your sweat glands are working overtime! And because you're beginning to perspire more, regular baths and underarm deodorants are newly important.

Your skin is becoming oily. Instead of just splashing water on your face every now and then, you need to care for your skin in special new ways to keep it clear and healthy.

You're approaching an age, too, when you're most likely to get cavities in your teeth and most likely to be wearing braces, which require some special care. Now that you're beginning to notice the opposite sex, having a nice smile and fresh breath probably means more to you than it did when you were just a little kid. Taking good care of your mouth and teeth can help you socially.

The fact is, it's cool to be clean and well-groomed. It'll make you look your very best. And it's healthy, too!

Cleanliness Is Cool!

How often should a person take a bath? How old should you be before using underarm deodorant? Also, once you have started your periods, what are the rules about baths or showers during that time? My grandma says that I shouldn't take any baths when I have my period. My mom says I should take even more baths than usual during that time. I'm all confused! ✻ GWEN P.

I keep hearing how uncircumcised boys need to wash themselves carefully, but what does that mean? What should I be doing?
✻ COLIN Q.

Daily baths or showers are an important part of any good grooming routine. Now that you're perspiring more and your skin has become oily, it's important to wash away that sweat and oil so you will always smell fresh and so the pores of your skin will not become clogged with dirt and oil.

Old wives' tales used to caution girls not to bathe during menstruation, and some people today, still feeling that menstruation is somehow unclean, advise girls to bathe even more during this time. The fact is, you just need to keep doing what you usually do—taking a daily bath or shower—whatever time of the month it is. If you really want to take an extra bath during your period or to cleanse your external genital area with a washcloth or special premoistened cleaning tissue between showers or baths, that's fine if it will make you feel more comfortable. But menstruation is *not* a hygienic emergency. It's simply part of your life.

The same is true if you're an uncircumcised male. You don't have to take more baths than anyone else. Just make sure, when you are bathing, to pull your foreskin back and clean the area underneath thoroughly.

Using an antiperspirant/deodorant should also become a part of your everyday grooming routine now that you're growing up. While

perspiration is a natural, necessary function that serves to cool your body and maintain a constant temperature, excessive perspiration can be controlled and body odor prevented by use of an antiperspirant/ deodorant. Those with aluminum chlorohydrate as the major, active ingredient are most effective.

When using a deodorant, read the instructions carefully. Often, for maximum protection, you should not apply it immediately after you come out of a steaming shower or hot bath. Your perspiration from that may simply wash the deodorant away. Instead, dry yourself thoroughly, cool down a bit and then apply the deodorant.

If you perspire a lot, you may feel like a freak. But the truth is, everyone perspires! And the more you worry about it, the more you may perspire! Also, it's important to know that you're more likely to perspire heavily at this time of your life as your body is adjusting to its many changes. As time goes on, you'll probably have less of a problem with excessive perspiration.

In the meantime, wear well-ventilated, absorbent clothes. A natural fabric such as cotton is especially good. Polyester and other man-made fabrics don't "breathe" well and can make you sweat more and can keep this sweat close to your body instead of helping it evaporate. Wear natural fabric shirts or blouses whenever you can.

Clean cotton is also a healthful choice for underwear. Your genital area needs air and ventilation so perspiration and natural secretions can evaporate instead of being trapped in the area, keeping the genitals moist and vulnerable to infections.

Girls should be aware of the fact that nylon underwear, tight jeans and pantyhose are not absorbent and can keep air away from the genital area, increasing the possibility of bacterial growth, yeast infections and odor. To help prevent this, choose cotton underwear or panties with a cotton crotch area. Take care to buy only those pantyhose having ventilated cotton crotches. And try to avoid wearing tight jeans for long periods of time.

If you're a girl, it's important to remember that, after urinating or defecating, you should wipe yourself from front to back so that you keep your genital area as free as possible of bacteria that is present in traces of fecal matter.

It's also a good idea to avoid sharing towels and washcloths or borrowing someone else's damp swimsuit. There are some vaginal infections that can be transmitted in that way.

Boys should be aware that "jock itch" (also called tinea cruris) can occur if one is not careful to wear clean underwear or, especially, a clean athletic supporter. A fungus can develop on a jockstrap that, moist with perspiration, is tossed into a gym locker and then used again without being washed. This fungus can cause an infection—an itchy, scaly rash—in the genital area. An over-the-counter drug called Tinactin will usually destroy this fungus. If more help is needed, your doctor can give you a very effective prescription medication. It's always better (and a lot less embarrassing) if you can just prevent this problem in the first place. You can do this by remembering to dry your body thoroughly after showering, bathing or working out and by always wearing clean cotton underwear and a freshly washed athletic supporter.

If you have sweaty feet, you need to give them special care in order to prevent athlete's foot. This fungal infection is most likely to happen to those whose feet are constantly hot and moist.

How do you keep your feet cool and healthy? Avoid wearing the same shoes—especially if these are rubbersoled, non-ventilated tennis or athletic shoes—day after day. Give your feet a break and wear a dry pair of shoes daily. In warm weather, wear sandals or go barefoot whenever you can. When you wear closed shoes, try to wear absorbent cotton socks. Whether or not that's possible, do wash your feet thoroughly every day and use talc or baby powder to keep them dry.

If you're in middle school and are changing clothes for gym class or showering afterward in a locker room—or if you regularly use a gym or health club facility locker room and shower—you can safeguard your foot health by wearing rubber shower sandals or swim socks. Plantar warts, usually found on the sole of the foot and picked up by a minor break in the skin in places like gym shower rooms, are very common in young teens. You decrease your risk of getting them by not going barefoot in gym showers. However, if you get a plantar wart, don't panic. These often disappear within a month. However, if it's painful (most likely if it's on your heel or the ball of your foot), check with your doctor to have it removed with liquid nitrogen or with an acid solution. Although there are some over-the-counter wart removers available, we don't advise these for plantar warts. If the wart isn't painful, leave it alone and wait for it to go away. If it's really bothering you, see your doctor.

Caring For Your Changing Skin

My mother says I have blackheads. What are they? Why do I have them? What can I do about them? I wash my face twice a day, but they're still there! ✻ AMBER L.

I have pimples on my face, especially my forehead. They seem to get worse just before my period. Why is that? What can I do? Should I go to a doctor? ✻ CATHY Y.

What can you do if you have zits on your back? Why would I get them there instead of just on my face? What can I do about this? ✻ JOHN D.

Most growing or nearly grown adolescents worry about their skin. And most report some skin problems around this time. A study from the National Center for Health Statistics revealed that only 27.7 percent of Americans between the ages of 12 and 17 have clear skin with no acne, lesions or scars.

So if you have blackheads or pimples, you have lots of company! But why are skin problems so common during this time of your life?

As we have seen, your hormone levels are increasing as your body begins to change and grow. These hormones cause the many oil glands in your skin (called sebaceous glands) to become more active. There are many of these glands on your face, back, chest and shoulders. As you mature, they begin to produce a fatty substance called *sebum*.

Sebum moves from the sebaceous gland to the opening of the skin, called the pore (see Figs. 7-1 to 7-3). It produces the oily skin so common in young people.

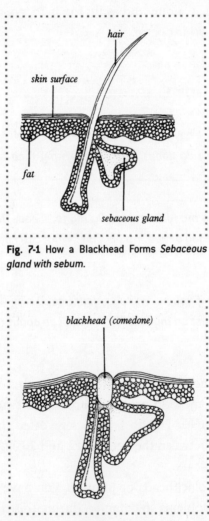

Fig. 7-1 How a Blackhead Forms *Sebaceous gland with sebum.*

Fig. 7-2 How a Blackhead Forms *Sebum and skin pigments form a blackhead.*

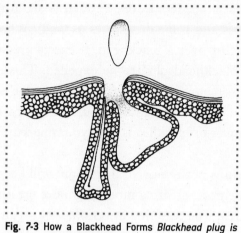

Fig. 7-3 How a Blackhead Forms *Blackhead plug is removed, unblocking the pore.*

But oily skin doesn't automatically mean that you'll have acne in the form of blackheads or pimples. It is only when your pore, the skin's passageway from the surface to the inner layers of your skin, becomes blocked with sebum that trouble starts.

When your pore is simply blocked with sebum, the result is a blackhead. Blackheads are *not* caused by dirt. Their dark color is caused by air mixing with sebum and skin pigments in your pore.

This plug of material is removed with a comedone extractor (Fig. 7-4). Your doctor can use this device to remove blackheads, or you can

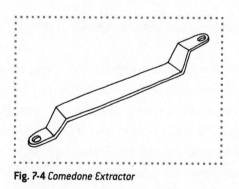

Fig. 7-4 *Comedone Extractor*

learn to use one at home (comedone extractors are available from surgical supply stores and some drugstores as well). When you press the comedone extractor over a blackhead, it exerts pressure on the skin and causes the blackhead plug to be expelled. This is the *only* way you should try to remove a blackhead. A comedone extractor should never be used on pimples because it could cause scarring. Picking or squeezing at pimples or blackheads with your fingertips can cause scarring, too.

If a blackhead is not removed, the sebum will keep building up in the gland and the pore, creating more and more pressure. Then bacteria invade the area. The resulting infection, which can cause red, pus-filled pimples, is what most people are talking about when they say they have acne. For some people, acne gets worse than pimples, progressing on to cysts that leave deep scars.

Heredity seems to have something to do with whether or not you will have acne and how severe it will be. If either of your parents had acne in their teens, you may have a problem with it, too.

But there are some things you can do to help keep your skin as clear as possible, whether or not you're genetically predisposed to acne.

■ Wash your face two or three times a day with ordinary soap or an antibacterial variety. This can help remove oil and bacteria from your skin and keep your pores open.

■ Wash your hair frequently, especially if it tends to be oily.

■ If you have blackheads, you might try using a pulverized soap to remove blackheads and open your pores. But be careful when you use it, because it can be very abrasive to your skin. Don't use it more than once or twice a day. And if you're black, don't use it at all. (Black skin tends to react to even slight irritation or injury by getting lighter or darker in patches. So it's important to be especially gentle to your skin.)

■ If you have acne in areas besides your face—your back or chest perhaps—be sure to wash these affected areas thoroughly as well. If you have acne on your back, use a back brush and an antibacterial and abrasive soap to scrub the area during your regular daily shower or bath.

■ After you've finished washing your face, rinse it in cold water to help close your pores again.

■ It can also help to use a cotton pad soaked in alcohol or an astringent to remove the last traces of dirt and oil. Don't overdo it with alcohol or other astringents, though. If your skin starts to feel dry, you're overdoing it. Your skin needs some oil to stay soft and healthy.

■ If (or when) you're allowed to wear makeup, avoid oil-based foundations. They can clog your pores. If acne is a problem for you, no makeup, or a medicated makeup and/or oil-free makeup, is a much better choice for you.

■ If your acne is mild, some over-the-counter acne lotions and creams may help dry out your skin just enough to help clear your complexion.

There are times and circumstances that can aggravate acne. Because a girl's hormone level is fluctuating just before her period, it's common to have an acne attack at that time.

Hot, humid weather and salty ocean water can also make acne worse. Be sure to wash your face frequently in the summer and rinse your face promptly with clear water after you come out of the surf.

It has not been scientifically established that either stress or particular foods (like chocolate) cause acne or make it worse. But some people do feel that certain foods seem to aggravate their acne. Some insist that they break out most during or just before stressful times—like exams or a first date. If this seems to be the case for you, avoid the foods you feel are a problem and give your skin extra care during rough times.

> *I have awful zits, and nothing I do makes any difference. Will I outgrow them? What can I do in the meantime? My skin looks terrible and I'm so embarrassed!* ❋ SCOTT Z.

If your acne doesn't get better with prescription gels or lotions, your doctor may give you some medication in pill form.

If you're a girl, your doctor may feel it's best to give you a prescription for birth control pills. These have been approved for use in treating acne as well as to prevent pregnancy. The hormone estrogen, which birth control pills always contain, seems to help control acne by suppressing oil gland secretions.

For those of either sex with very severe, cystic acne that hasn't been improved by other forms of treatment, treatment with Accutane (13-*cis*-retinoic acid) might be helpful. It is taken in pill form for eight weeks. Then the patient goes off it for eight weeks, then starts taking it again for another eight weeks if his or her doctor decides this is necessary. Many people have found that their skin continues to improve even after they stop taking Accutane.

This powerful drug has some troublesome side effects, so it is generally used only in severe cases and then only under the careful supervision of a dermatologist.

The most common side effect of Accutane is severe drying and chapping of the lips. However, more serious side effects include a rise in cholesterol levels and some cases of depression, psychosis or even suicidal behavior while taking this drug. However, despite all the publicity that this particular side effect has received, it isn't yet known whether Accutane may make existing depression—which a teen may have for other reasons—worse or whether it can cause depression. Obviously, if you're taking Accutane and start to feel depressed, let your doctor know right away!

Another serious side effect of Accutane makes it very important for any girl being treated with this drug to avoid pregnancy. Accutane can cause devastating birth defects in babies conceived while their mothers were taking the drug. Medical experts are so concerned about this that it is suggested that any young woman, even those who are virgins and fully expect to stay that way until they're older, should take birth control pills along with Accutane so they're protected against an unintended pregnancy that could happen, for example, in case they may be raped. *That's* how concerned doctors are about the terrible birth defects that this drug can cause. (This danger of having a baby with such birth defects is only present if you get pregnant when actually taking Accutane, not in the weeks, months and years *after* you finished using it.)

Needless to say, Accutane is not something you take if you have a few zits. It's only for really severe cases of acne.

I heard that sunbathing can give you cancer. Is that true? I love to go to the beach and spend lots of time outdoors. How can I keep from getting cancer? ✷ TERRI T.

Suntans are a seasonal fad year after year. A recent survey of more than 10,000 teens nationwide revealed that 89 percent of girls and 78 percent of boys said that most of their friends actively work on getting and keeping great tans.

But this tanning trend is a dangerous one. Longtime overexposure to the sun's ultraviolet rays puts you at risk for skin cancers, including the potentially deadly malignant melanoma. And the biggest risk factors for this cancer occur not simply over time, but as a result of serious sunburns and prolonged sun exposure right now—in your childhood and teenage years!

This doesn't mean that you can't enjoy outdoor activities or hit the beach regularly. It simply means that seeking a suntan is not a healthy move.

What can you do to have fun in the sun and protect your skin at the same time?

■ Use a sunscreen! It's especially important to use one with high blocking power early in the season when your skin is unaccustomed to lots of sun exposure. Buy a sunscreen that has the following ingredients listed on its label: zinc oxide and titanium dioxide. These are physical sun blockers that deflect light off the skin's surface and are also kind to sensitive skin. While suncreens have had numerical ratings of sun protection factors—numbers like 15 or 30 or 45—the Federal Drug Administration's ratings now range from "minimum" protection (if they have a sun protection factor of 2 to 11), "moderate" (for SPF 12–29) or "high" for an SPF over 30.

■ Slather it on! Use about a half-teaspoon of sunscreen on each arm and also on your face and neck. For each leg, your back, chest and stomach, use even more: a whole teaspoon or more on each exposed part. And reapply this every hour or two while you're in the sun. Even waterproof sunscreens lose their effectiveness after an hour or so, especially when you're in the water or sweating a lot on a hot summer day.

■ Try to stay out of the sun when its rays are most powerful and direct—usually between 10 A.M. and 3 P.M. If you must be outdoors during those hours, stay in the shade, or take a beach umbrella or a totable open tent to the beach or park.

■ If you're a swimmer, you need sunscreen, too. Water doesn't shield you from the sun's ultraviolet rays. So apply sunscreen both before and after swimming.

■ Don't expect clouds or a light beach cover-up to protect you. Ultraviolet rays can penetrate both and you could end up with quite a sunburn. Use sunscreen no matter what you're wearing and whatever the weather! Wear a hat (you *can* find a cool-looking one if you really look) to protect your face and a shirt to cover your shoulders, back and chest. There are even some shirts and cover-ups that are made to be somewhat sunscreening. There is also a new spray, applied to regular clothing that can supposedly help protect you from harmful sun exposure. However, we have no definite information at this time about whether or how well that spray actually works. So keep covered and apply that sunscreen!

■ Put extra sunscreen on your nose, lips, shoulders and knees—places most likely to get sunburned.

■ Apply a moisturizer to your skin after you come in from spending a lot of time in the sun. This will help keep your skin soft.

■ If you do get a sunburn, putting cool, wet washcloths or towels on your skin can help. Soothing lotions for sunburn and aspirin or aspirin-substitutes can also ease your discomfort.

■ If your sunburn is severe, see your doctor for prescription medicines that can ease your pain and reduce the swelling that severe burns can cause.

■ Avoid tanning salons!! A recent survey found that 14 percent of young adolescent girls had used a tanning bed at a salon in the past year. This has the same dangers as lying in the sun. It can even be more dangerous because most people don't take the precautions in tanning beds that they do on the beach. After all, if you're paying good money to get tanned in a salon, you're not likely to bring along the sunscreen! So don't even go there. Save your money, your skin and your health.

■ Be especially careful if you're taking medications like ibuprofen, tetracycline, birth control pills or other drugs that your doctor may warn you can increase your sensitivity to the sun and tendency to sunburn.

Why are we making such a fuss about something as simple as sunbathing? Because the damage to your skin can be a lot more serious than a painful sunburn now or wrinkles when you're older. Overexposure to sun and, especially, several serious sunburns in childhood or adolescence can put you at serious risk for the deadliest of skin cancers: malignant melanoma. Unfortunately, this isn't something you only get when you're old. Melanoma can happen in young people, too. A friend of ours named Sandi was a beach-loving blue-eyed blonde who got sunburned a lot between her summer tans when she was in junior high and high school. Sandi was diagnosed with melanoma in her senior year of college—when she was just 21 years old. She died a few years later.

Unfortunately, Sandi is not an especially unusual case. Studies show that the rate of melanoma in young women has increased some 60 percent among young women ages 15 to 29 in the last few decades.

So slather on that sunscreen! You can still have fun in the sun. But just use common sense.

Removing Unwanted Hair

What does it mean if you have some hair on your face—like sideburns, sort of—and you're a girl? How can a person get rid of hair like this? ✻ GINA C.

Is it true that if you shave your legs, the hair grows back heavier? That's what my mother keeps telling me, and that's why she doesn't want me to shave my legs until I'm in high school. I'm in the sixth grade and I have heavy, really black, ugly hair all over my legs and the boys tease me constantly! Would it hurt to shave now? ✻ SHARON W.

When should a boy start shaving? What kind of razor is best to use? The reason I'm asking is that when my older brother started shaving, his acne seemed to get worse and his skin was always really sore. I have the beginnings of acne already and, even though I don't need to shave yet, I'd like some information about how to avoid going through the trouble my brother is going through. ❋ GREG M.

Although hair growth under the arms, on the forearms and on the legs is a normal part of growing up for both sexes, many girls choose to remove what they feel is excess hair, particularly underarm and leg hair. It is not uncommon for some girls to have some facial hair as well. This is particularly likely if your ancestors came from a Mediterranean country (Italy, Greece or anywhere in the Middle East). Many of these girls are anxious to remove traces of unwanted facial hair.

A minority of girls may not develop excess hair on the face until their late teens, when its sudden appearance can signal a hormone imbalance or glandular problem. In such cases, treatment from a physician is necessary.

Boys usually don't start to think about hair removal—usually in the form of shaving their faces—until they're in their mid- or late teens. That, too, is optional. But most boys do choose to shave.

How old do you have to be to remove excess hair? When you're old enough to have the hair that troubles you. If your parents disagree, try to talk it over calmly. Explain to them how you feel. It *isn't* true, by the way, that shaving or otherwise removing hair makes it grow back thicker. You may feel it more as it's starting its regrowth, but that's just because you're feeling the cut ends of the hair.

What are the best ways to remove unwanted hair? Many girls prefer to remove facial hair with a hair-removal cream called a depilatory. These chemical hair removers dissolve hair at the skin surface but do not remove hair permanently. Some girls use them on their legs and underarms and may use special facial formulas for facial hair.

Some girls choose to permanently remove facial hair with electrolysis. This is a somewhat expensive, time-consuming and uncomfortable procedure that must be done by a professional. A tiny electrode, which enters the hair follicle via a needle, destroys the hair root with a high-speed electric current. If you are considering electrolysis, ask your doctor for a referral to an experienced technician.

Removing excess hair with hot wax—a procedure called "waxing"—does not remove hair permanently, but can get rid of it for a longer period than shaving or chemical hair removers and may discourage some regrowth of hair. Hot wax is applied to the area, allowed to cool and then pulled off, taking the excess hair with it. As you might have guessed, this is not entirely pain-free, and even though there are kits you can use at home, it's best to have waxing done by a professional in a beauty salon or special waxing studio.

Most people who want to remove excess hair, however, shave it off. Most girls shave their underarms and legs; most boys shave their faces. Here are some ideas for safe, effective shaving:

■ A blade razor will usually give you a closer shave and tends to be less irritating if you have acne. An electric razor does not protect you from cuts and can cause razor burns or rash. However, an electric razor can be a good choice if the skin in the area you're shaving is very dry. Another plus is that electric razors remove less oil from the skin.

■ Be sure to moisturize the area to be shaved before you start shaving. Soaking in a hot tub or taking a hot shower for several minutes before you begin to shave can help get your skin ready. So can washing your skin with soap and/or using a shaving cream or electric pre-shave lotion.

■ Shave in the direction of the hair growth, not against it. This will help to prevent skin irritation, particularly if you have acne or your skin is sore or sunburned.

■ If you have acne, use a blade razor rather than an electric one. This is much less likely to cause further irritation and scarring.

■ You're more likely to cut yourself when you're inexperienced and/or when you're in a rush. Take time to shave in slow, even strokes. And take comfort in the fact that, as you acquire more skill and confidence, you're less likely to nick yourself with the razor. In the meantime, a styptic pencil, available in drugstores, can help stop the bleeding quickly.

■ There are no set rules about how often you should shave. People have different rates of hair regrowth. Some people, quite often those whose ancestors came from Scandinavian countries or Asia, need to shave much less often than others.

Most men, once they are fully grown and mature, shave their faces almost every day. A study for the Gillette Company found that most adult men shave about five times a week, with younger men in their late teens usually shaving less often than that.

Women vary greatly in how often they need to shave their legs or underarms. Some do it every day. Others need to shave only once every few weeks.

For women whose excess hair appears due to a hormonal imbalance, a physician may be able to help by treating her with one of several prescription drugs.

Hand And Nail Care

There's a girl at school that I like, but she told me she didn't like me because my fingernails gross her out. What am I supposed to do? Men don't do their nails! How do men take care of their nails without looking too . . . feminine? ✳ PETE K.

Could you tell me how to do a manicure? Some girls in my class have really nice hands and nails. Mine look awful. My hands are chapped a lot, especially in the winter. And my nails aren't nice-looking at all. I'm embarrassed to ask anyone I know to show me how to make my nails look pretty. And my mother doesn't care about stuff like that so I can't ask her. The only thing she says is that I can't use nail polish, even the clear kind, because I'm 10 and she says that's too young.

✳ JENNIFER A.

Keeping your hands clean, healthy and well groomed is vital whether you're male or female. If the skin on your hands is dry and chapped—this is especially likely in the winter, if you do dishes a lot or if you have a hobby such as pottery or developing photos that requires you to keep your hands wet a lot—use hand cream, even if you're a boy. It's not sissy stuff! It's necessary to replace some of the moisture and oils that water and cold weather take away. If your hands are severely dry or chapped, cover them with hand cream and then cotton gloves that are made to be worn while you sleep. Drug and five-and-dime stores often carry these.

Clean nails are attractive—and something others notice more than you realize. Take time every day or so to clean underneath your nails and to scrub them with a special nail brush and warm, soapy water.

If you're a boy, keep your nails clean and neatly clipped (see Fig. 7-5). It also isn't sissy stuff to file the rough edges with an emery board. If your nails chip and break a lot, it could be due to dryness or bad habits. For example, do you drum your nails on hard surfaces (like a desk), bite them or pick at things with them?

If you're a girl, do you use lots of nail polish (clear or otherwise) and remover? The chemicals in these, used frequently, can cause nail dryness. If your nails are dry, it can help to soak them in warm olive oil or baby oil and then use a hand lotion that has a lanolin base. You should also think twice before using artificial nails. These can cause allergic reactions and/or fungal infections. If you take time to care for your nails, you can have pretty and completely natural nails!

How do you give yourself a manicure? Here's what you will need:

a small bowl of warm water, or warm water mixed with baby shampoo and baby oil (or olive oil)

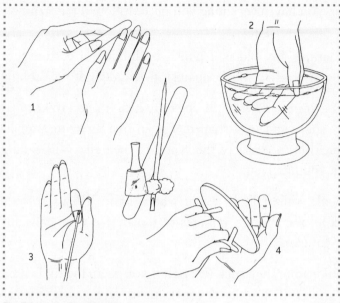

Fig. 7-5 How to Do a Manicure

1. File dry nails in one direction, from sides to center.

2. Soak nails in warm water mixed with baby shampoo and baby (or olive) oil.

3. Push cuticles back with orange stick.

4. Buff nails to a healthy shine.

an emery board

an orange stick

cotton

baby oil or olive oil

hand lotion

Optional:

buffer and buffing paste

clear nail polish

nail polish remover

When you have everything you need, follow these steps:

1. Remove any old nail polish by holding a cotton pad soaked with nail polish remover against it. Avoid vigorous rubbing.

2. File your nails with the emery board. It's best to keep your nails fairly short and oval-shaped. File in one direction, not back and forth, from the sides to the center of the nail. Nails should be dry when you file them.

3. Soak your nails in warm water (or in the water/shampoo/oil mixture) for about 5 minutes to moisturize your nails and soften your cuticles.

4. Take an orange stick (it's best if you wrap the tip in a bit of cotton) and gently push back your cuticles. *Don't* use a cuticle remover or try to cut the cuticle with scissors! Just push it back very gently.

5. Put lots of hand cream on your hands and work it into every part of your hand, including all your fingers.

6. Wash your hands and use a nail brush dipped in soapy water to clean any dirt or hand cream from underneath or around your nails.

That's the end of the basic manicure. That's all there is to it! If you want to add some extra gloss to your nails, you might try the following:

■ If you aren't allowed to use clear nail polish or don't like polish, you can buff your nails to a pretty shine. To do this, you need a buffer (see Fig. 7-5) and some buffing paste. Put a little of this paste on each nail and then buff gently for a healthy-looking shine.

■ If you are allowed to use polish, apply three thin coats (rather than one thick one) to your nails, starting with your little finger. Try to put the polish on the center of the nail first and then fill in the sides. If you get some on your skin, just take an orange stick with cotton on the tip or a Q-Tip dipped in nail polish remover and gently rub it off. You might want to put on a glossy top coat after your last coat of polish has dried.

If you do wear nail polish, try to repair chips in the polish by just filling in the chips instead of doing the whole nail over. Again, using too much nail polish remover can be drying to your nails.

Caring For Your Hair

My best friend says that if you wash your hair more than once or twice a week, it will fall out. My problem is, I have very oily hair and if I wash it only once a week, it looks stringy and terrible. Last week, I washed it three times in one week, and when I finished washing it the last time, I noticed some hairs in the sink. Could I really get bald from washing my hair too much? ✳ BETHANY B.

My hair is really dull and hard to control. It never looks right. What can I do? ✳ EMILY H.

The best way to care for your hair is to keep it clean and conditioned.

There is *no* harm in washing your hair several times a week or even every day. Many people wash their hair every day with a mild shampoo and conditioner. Frequent shampooing removes excess oil from your hair and scalp. Your hair will have more body and, with conditioner, more luster.

Be careful, though, not to damage your hair with too-frequent permanents or prolonged sessions with a hot blow-dryer. If your hair tends to be dry, use a conditioner made especially for dry hair and use the blow-dryer sparingly. You might use it just to style your wet hair and then, when your hair is in place but still damp, turn it off and let your hair air dry naturally. Some women get wash-and-wear haircuts that allow them to skip blow-drying at least some of the time.

A good haircut is a must if you have hard-to-manage hair. This is true for boys as well as girls. There are a lot of new haircutting and styling salons that will give you a good basic haircut at low cost. A good haircut in a style that's becoming to you can help tame even the most unmanageable locks.

If you notice that you lose hair during or after a shampoo or when you brush your hair, don't panic. It's normal to lose some amount of hair every day.

Why? Because hair follicles have both active and resting cycles. After growing a hair for several years, the follicle will shed that hair and rest for a few months. This takes place constantly, and most of the time your hair loss is not noticeable when you look at your hair or scalp.

There are some instances, however, when your hair follicles will shed their hair prematurely and the loss will be quite noticeable. Most often, this happens when something unusual is happening to you physically. For example, if you have had a dramatic weight loss and/or are suffering from an eating disorder such as anorexia nervosa you may have some hair loss. Other serious disorders (among them hypothyroidism), some anti-cancer drugs, scalp allergies to beauty products or scalp infections—all can cause hair loss. If you seem to be losing more hair than usual, it's a good idea to see your physician for a checkup to make sure that all is well.

If your hair looks dull and lifeless, it could be due to dryness or to overuse of certain hair products, such as hair spray or styling gel. Or it could be because you didn't rinse the shampoo and conditioner out of it completely the last time you washed it. Dirt and air pollution can also take the shine out of your hair. You can put the shine back in by shampooing frequently and then rinsing your hair thoroughly.

Eating the right foods and getting plenty of vitamins can also make your hair shine. Dull hair, in fact, may be a clue that you lack vitamin B_{12} and need to eat more eggs, milk, fish and lean meat to start looking your best!

Thinking About Piercings And Tattoos

I'm almost 12 and want to get my ears pierced but my parents are against it. They said I could get an infection, and my mom thinks people can even get AIDS that way. How can I convince her that all my friends already have pierced ears and nothing bad happened to them?! ✳ EMILY R.

I really, really want two things before I start eighth grade next month: my naval pierced (which looks soooo cool!) and a small tattoo. My parents are freaking out and won't let me. What can I do? ✳ ASHLEIGH S.

Although ear piercing has been popular among teens for some years now and is generally safe if performed properly under antiseptic conditions, piercing other body parts and getting tattoos can be a problem.

If you just want to get your earlobes pierced, that's fine, especially if you have your ears pierced by a physician using sterile equipment. Some jewelry and department stores have trained technicians who perform ear piercing. Usually, they pierce the earlobe with the sterilized post of the earring itself. This is safe if your earlobe is sterilized with alcohol before and after the piercing and if the earring post itself is sterile and has never been used by another person. Post earrings are usually worn continuously for about six weeks while the earlobes heal. If the technician is using a piercing gun, go elsewhere! This device can't be sterilized properly and may put you at risk for any number of blood-borne infections including HIV and several types of hepatitis.

Ear piercing is not a do-it-yourself project with a friend wielding a sewing needle. The chance of infection is too great. Have the piercing done by a professional—preferably a doctor or, at the very least, a trained technician. And follow a careful routine while your ears are healing. Dab your lobes regularly with alcohol or mild soap and always dip your earrings in alcohol before inserting them. Also, while your ears are healing from the piercing, don't remove or change your earrings.

Recently, other body piercings—from eyebrow to nose, lips to tongue, navel to multiple studs in the upper ear—as well as tattoos, have become trendy among teens. All of these can be problematic. Body piercing carries considerable risk of infection and can also be quite painful. The risk of infection is especially great when piercing is done in the tongue, the lips and the inside the mouth. Also, metal in the mouth can damage teeth. Swelling of the pierced tongue can make breathing, speaking and eating much more difficult. If you're determined to get body piercing anyway, get it done by a doctor under sterile conditions. That way, your risk of infection is less. Better still, find another, less painful way to look cool.

We might say the same about tattoos. These are definitely teen trends: 10 to 13 percent of teens 12 to 18 have tattoos, compared to 3 to 8 percent of the general population, and girls are more likely than boys to get them. There are a couple of problems with tattoos: You risk infection if the tattooing is not done under sterile conditions, including infection with the HIV virus or hepatitis B and C; and tattoos may brand you as a wild child—someone who might be into drugs, gangs or sex—a reputation you may not want to have for a lot of reasons; and tattoos can't just be washed away when you get tired of them, break up with a person whose name is immortalized on your body or grow out of wanting to look trendy and want to look properly professional for job-hunting. While tattoos can be removed now by laser, this process is painful and costs about $1,200 to $1,500.

If you're determined to get a tattoo anyway, here are a few more realities to consider. First, at the very least, you will need your parents' permission to get a tattoo. That is the law in many states. In still other states, the tattooing of minors under the age of 18 is illegal under any circumstances. Don't be tempted to go the informal route and have a friend give you an amateur tattoo. Chances are, it won't look good and your risk of infection will be greater. If you can legally get a tattoo and your parents give their permission, go to a tattoo parlor that is clean and where gloves and sterilized needles are used. That will decrease your risk of infection.

An even better idea: Instead of something permanent, give yourself the chance to change your mind (and to look trendy without having to check out state laws or ask your parents' permission) and try temporary tattoos—the herbal variety that is applied with a brush or plastic cone and lasts two to four weeks or the press-on type. You can have all the fun of shocking your parents and looking cool without having to live with the same old tattoo forever or going through a painful removal process.

Tips For Good Dental Health

Help! I have lots of cavities in my teeth even though I don't eat all that much candy. What can I do to stop getting so many cavities? I REALLY HATE going to the dentist! ✻ MARK C.

People tell me I have bad breath. How can I have bad breath when I brush my teeth twice a day and use mouthwash? ✻ SARA N.

I just recently got braces and my dentist told me I shouldn't eat sweets at all. Why can't I? I don't have any fillings! Why should braces make any difference? ✻ DAVID H.

Caring for your teeth is important because dental health is part of your overall health and well-being—and a healthy mouth also means fresh breath and a nice smile.

It's especially important to take good care of your teeth now because now is when many young people begin to have dental problems. Some preteens and young teenagers notice that they have more cavities now than ever before. Often this happens because you're eating on the run and are too busy to brush your teeth after every meal. You may also be eating a lot of junk foods or fast foods. Many of these foods, from ready-to-eat cereals and frozen dinners to fast-food French fries, have a lot of sugar in them. Much of the sugar you eat, especially if you're not an avid candy fan, can come from these "hidden sugars."

Sugar can lead to a buildup of harmful bacteria on the teeth. The combination of sugar and bacteria causes plaque, a film that sticks to the teeth and that can lead to tooth decay and gum irritation and disease.

It is gum disease, called periodontal disease, even more than tooth decay that can give you serious dental problems later on in life and persistent bad breath even now. Gum disease develops when plaque gets below the gum line and causes your gums to get irritated and inflamed. If your gums bleed easily, especially when you're brushing your teeth, you may have early-stage gum disease called gingivitis.

What can you do to protect your teeth and gums?

■ Brush your teeth with a soft-bristled toothbrush after every meal and floss between your teeth at least once a day or, preferably, after every meal. If you're unable to brush and floss after a meal out, rinsing your mouth with water immediately after eating can help.

This daily care can make a huge difference in your dental health. One dentist told us that when she was a child and teenager, her father (also a dentist) absolutely insisted that she carry a toothbrush and dental floss to school with her so she could clean her teeth thoroughly after lunch. She says there were times when she thought it was a lot of trouble and was afraid her classmates would notice and make fun of her. But she was rewarded for her trouble with perfect teeth and wonderful dental health. She is now in her thirties and has yet to get a single cavity!

It doesn't have to take you a lot of time to care for your teeth every day. A thorough brushing takes only a few minutes. And you can always floss your teeth while watching TV or listening to the radio or stereo—things you would normally do anyway. Flossing is really easy (see Fig. 7-6) and takes no time at all. It can be very important not only for your dental health, but also for your general health. As strange as it sounds, people who don't take care of their teeth and gums by brushing and flossing are at greater risk for infections that can get into the bloodstream from the diseased

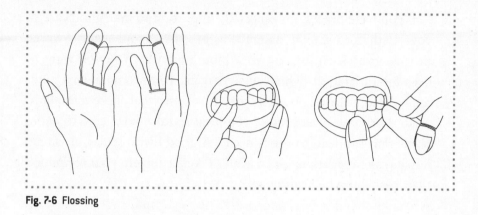

Fig. 7-6 Flossing

gums and can damage your heart. So flossing is a quick and easy way to safeguard your health as well as your smile!

■ If your teeth are very crowded and you find it's hard to reach your back molars with your toothbrush, get a smaller, child-size toothbrush for your back teeth. Using a Water Pik can also help you get food particles out of those tight, hard-to-reach areas of your mouth.

It's especially important, if your 12-year molars or wisdom teeth are coming in but are still partially covered by gum tissue, to rinse those areas with warm water to make sure that food particles don't get trapped underneath the gum to cause tooth decay or infections. If you do get a slight infection—swelling or irritation in the gums around an emerging tooth—rinse the area repeatedly with warm water that has been mixed with salt. If that doesn't help, be sure to see your dentist.

■ Eat foods that promote good dental health: fruit, crunchy raw vegetables, salads and protein-rich snacks. This doesn't mean you can't ever have any of your old favorites—like sweets or fast food—but the more healthy variety you have in your diet and the more nutritious, fiber-rich food you eat, the better your overall health will be!

■ If you have braces, it's especially important to take good care of your teeth. You should, as much as possible, avoid sugary sweets. Because braces can irritate your mouth anyway, you will want to keep gum irritation (which sugary snacks can promote) to a minimum. Also, because your teeth may be somewhat more difficult to clean when you have braces, you need to take extra care to avoid foods that can lead to tooth decay. A good diet, regular brushing, flossing and irrigation with a Water Pik can all help your teeth look their best—and be healthy, too!

■ Visit your dentist regularly, preferably twice a year, to get a checkup and to have your teeth professionally cleaned. Professional cleaning is essential to remove all traces of plaque, including whatever might be below your gum line.

Going to the dentist doesn't have to be an ordeal if you take good care of your teeth in the ways we've described and if you see him or her regularly instead of just when you have serious problems. Good preventive care can help you to have—and keep—a great smile!

In fact, taking good care of your changing body—from your head to your toes—will help you to look and feel your very best.

8

Your Changing Feelings

I'm almost 12 and am moody a lot. I cry a lot without knowing why. I feel alone at times, even though I'm really not. My parents are pretty decent, my older brother treats me O.K. and we have a nice house and clothes and things like that. I also have some good friends. So why am I so moody all of a sudden? ✳ KIM W.

I get mad at my mother over the smallest things. It's like she can't do anything right. We used to be real close, but now we fight all the time. She says I've changed. But she really upsets me and embarrasses me in front of my friends by treating me like I was a baby instead of a sixth grader! What's happening? Is this normal? How can I get her to stop treating me like a baby? ✳ DANIELLE F.

I'm in love with my math teacher—even though he gave me a C last semester. He's 26 and just perfect: really handsome, fun and nice. Even though he's married and his wife is going to have a baby this summer, I keep dreaming about him being in love with me. I can't get him out of my mind. I know I'll never meet anyone else like him. What should I do? Should I tell him how I feel about him? I'm only 11, so most people would think this is dumb, but I really, really love him! ✳ ALEXA M.

As you grow and change, you'll have many new feelings. There is the stress that the rapid changes in your life can bring. And there is the new push for independence as you suddenly find yourself arguing or finding fault with your parents.

You may be feeling moody a lot: happy one minute and really depressed and upset the next—and all the time not quite knowing why. You may have new loves in your life: special friends and teachers or popular stars you love and admire. And you may be wondering who you are—and who you're growing to be.

If you've had *any* of these feelings, you're normal! They're all a part of changing from child to young adult.

The Stress Of Change

I'm really down a lot because I feel ugly. When I was a kid, I felt pretty good about my body, but now that it's changing and I've gained some weight, I feel really ugly and am scared that no one will like me when I start junior high this fall. ✳ DIANA J.

Until this year, I did really well in school. But now everything is horrible. I'm in seventh grade and hate junior high! I don't have any real friends, and I don't know most of my teachers very well. I hate going to a big school. I miss my old one where I knew everybody. Don't tell me things will get better because I've been here two months already and it just stays horrible! ✳ CHRIS A.

What can you do if no one wants to be your friend? I don't have anyone to eat lunch with even. I don't know whether it's because I'm shorter than most of the other guys, or whether it's because my family just

moved here so I'm new in school, or whether it's something else, but I
feel sort of lost without a friend. ✷ MATTHEW S.

Stress happens a lot during these growing years. That's probably no news to you. For a lot of people, middle school or junior high is absolutely the pits. For others, the biggest stress is feeling different from the person you used to be and from your friends and classmates as well. Recent studies have shown that girls who are early bloomers show the most stress and depression during this time. That could be because, having put on the weight that normally comes with physical maturing (or being a bit overweight to begin with), they feel uncomfortable and ashamed that their bodies aren't as slim as those of their later-developing classmates. Because they look older than they really are, more may be expected of them. And boys have been known to tease early-developing girls nonstop about the changes that are obvious. And some girls feel stress because they get attention from older boys and don't always know how to handle this. Studies have shown that early-maturing girls who also date at an earlier age than most tend to be most at risk for serious dieting and eating disorders and depression. It isn't the contact with boys that is the problem. It is, quite possibly, facing the new experience of romantic relationships before being quite able to handle the experience emotionally. Interestingly enough, the same studies have shown that girls who have boys as *friends* are less likely than any other young teen group to be depressed or stressed out.

So if it seems that you have lots of male *friends* but no real boyfriend, this is an advantage—at least in terms of your mental health right now. (The same is true for boys, too: Girls who are friends may be more likely to listen and show support than some male friends who joke around and tease to bring a guy up when he's feeling down.)

But many young people feel stressed out because they feel no one could understand them. They feel different in so many ways.

If that describes you, take heart! This feeling isn't forever. Probably at no other time in your life will there be so much diversity in the way people of the same age look. One 12-year-old may look like a child, another like a young adult. There may be some huge differences in height and level of physical maturity between you and many of your classmates. And, wherever you are in this wide range of normal, you will probably have times of feeling different, times when you wonder if you really are normal.

If it's any comfort, "Am I normal?" is the question we've been asked most frequently by both preteens and teenagers. It can help to read everything you can about growing up and development. It can also help to talk to others—friends you especially trust, parents, relatives, your school nurse, your physician. They may be able to reassure you and, in the case of friends, let you know that you're not the only one who worries about being normal and attractive. It's very common to feel different at this time in your life. But if you can reach out to others, you will find that you're not quite as different as you thought and you're definitely *not* alone!

Another major stress at this time in your life is changing schools. Lots of young people change schools frequently due to family moves, and that can be very difficult, especially at a time when friends are becoming more and more important to you.

One of the toughest school adjustments can be the move everyone makes from elementary school to junior high. You go from the personal atmosphere of a neighborhood elementary school where you know most of the kids and have one teacher to the larger campus of a junior high where most people are, at least initially, strangers to you and where you walk from class to class, having different teachers for each subject.

In junior high, too, a lot more seems to be expected of you. Teachers demand more. Parents start talking about the importance of your making decent grades so you can get into college or a good job training program. And social life is different, too: Boys and girls are beginning to see each other in a new way. There are dances and other co-ed social activities. Suddenly, being popular with the opposite sex may be much more important to you than it used to be. And lack of popularity can hurt a lot.

That brings us to another common stress at this time: worrying about being liked and accepted and having friends. At this time in your life you have a new need for friends to share feelings and experiences with and help you feel that you're normal.

This is a time when you need friendship the most. But it isn't easy to make friends. It isn't always easy to feel accepted. This is a time when, because of their own insecurities and worries about being normal, your classmates can be very critical and intolerant of differences.

It's a lot of change to handle at once. It's easy to feel left out, unloved and unlovable, like a number rather than a person and overwhelmed by all that's expected of you. How do you begin to cope with all this change?

■ **Start small.** It takes time to get used to these big changes in your life. It takes time to make new friends and feel comfortable with new ways of socializing. Tackle one challenge at a time, and do some small thing every day to help yourself adjust.

This may mean saying "Hi" to one or two new people a day.

It may mean joining a school club or activity where you can meet others who share some of your interests.

Or it may mean making friends with someone of the opposite sex and getting more comfortable with a boy or girl as a person and a good friend before you begin to think seriously of dates.

Any major challenge—from adjusting to junior high to cleaning your room—can seem overwhelming at first. But if you can break it down into little pieces—turning a few strangers into acquaintances and then friends; getting to know a small group of people who share your interests; or becoming comfortable just talking to someone of the opposite sex for a while—you can get a start in adjusting to your new life circumstances. And each small start can make a big difference!

■ **Get organized.** This can help in a lot of ways. If you're feeling overwhelmed by increased homework, harder courses or the expectations others have of you, you can take some of the stress off yourself by approaching these problems in an organized way. Now is a good time to learn how to budget your time so you can get homework out of the way and leave time to do fun things, too. Now is a good time to decide which courses are hard for you and give yourself extra time to study for and maybe get extra help with those. Making up your own time schedule can help you get things done more effectively. When you fulfill your obligations, from homework to household chores, others are less likely to tell you what to do with the rest of your time. You'll have more freedom to choose what you like!

Decide what are the activities you really like and want to do from day to day. Decide how you really want to spend your free time. That way, you can organize your thoughts and express your wishes clearly if someone asks you what you want to do. This will help others—from parents to friends—know you better. It can also help in getting them to stop making so many decisions for you. There are times when you will agree with and want to go along with your parents or friends. But when you disagree and have other ideas, it helps to know exactly how you feel and express this to others clearly and calmly. This is one of the ways you grow to become your own person.

■ **Exercise regularly.** When you're tense, anxious and under stress, regular, vigorous exercise can help you calm down. It can also help ease depression, if you've been feeling a bit low about school or your social life. And, of course, exercise does wonderful things for your health and looks, too.

Taking up a new sport or an active hobby (like any form of dancing) can also help you begin to feel more comfortable with your changing body.

■ **Give yourself a break.** Don't expect too much too soon. It isn't possible to have everyone in your new school like you. Some people, for reasons that may have little to do with you personally, will always be indifferent to you and maybe even dislike you. That doesn't mean you're not a likable, lovable, worthwhile person. Don't expect instant friendships. Trust and caring take time to grow. But a good friendship is worth taking time to build!

If you're upset because you're having trouble with the changes of junior high, give yourself time. Eventually, it will all seem normal—dashing from class to class, having five, six or seven different teachers and, possibly, hundreds of classmates. Some people may seem to adjust right away. But it usually takes several months for most to start to feel comfortable in such a new and different setting.

Until you begin to feel more at ease, do at least two or three things every day that help you to relax. Maybe this means listening to your favorite music for half an hour before you go to bed. Maybe it means talking to someone who loves and cares about you. Maybe it means a walk in the park, a stroll on the beach or just walking or riding your bike around the neighborhood. Maybe it means curling up on your bed with your favorite cat or dog and just petting him or her for a while. (Experts have noted that petting a favorite animal can help calm you when you're under stress or upset.) In short, do something that brings you pleasure at least several times a day. This can help a lot if you're worried or upset about other areas of your life. Pleasurable interludes can be ways of giving yourself little vacations to help you have more energy and feel better. They can bring some familiar comforts to your life when so many other things are changing.

Living With A Changing Family

I feel like the life I have always known is over because my parents just told me they're getting a divorce! They said they've thought about it for a long time and just waited until I was old enough to understand and take care of myself more. But I'm not! I'm only 13, and I don't understand! And I feel like somehow it's my fault. Maybe if I didn't try to act grown-up, maybe if I were more immature, they wouldn't be getting a divorce. How can I convince them that I need them both and want things to be like they were before? ✳ CHEYENNE W.

I'm sort of down because my brother Ryan left for college back east last week and now it's just me and my parents and things don't seem right. I guess you could say I really miss him and am scared that nothing will ever be the same. What if he changes so much at college that he won't want to hang out with me next summer? ✳ BRAD O.

Just about the time you have about as many changes as you can handle, your family starts changing. Maybe this means that an older brother or sister goes away to college or joins the armed services or gets married—and you wonder if you can stay close with all the miles and life differences between you. Or this might mean that your mom, who has taken time off her career to see you through to increased independence, decides to go back to work—or family circumstances (like college coming up fast for you and your siblings or a strained family budget) require that she work full-time now—and you're left to fend for yourself and find that you aren't quite as independent yet as you thought. Or your parents may have made the painful decision to divorce—and, like Cheyenne's parents—they have this idea you should be able to handle it all just fine now that you're nearly grown-up.

Except you're not so sure. As you go through all the physical, emotional and school changes you're facing right now, you may feel the need for a secure home and family more than ever (even though it's hard to admit this most days!).

So how can you handle it when your family starts changing just about the time *you* need everyone and everything around you to stay the same?

■ **Allow your feelings to happen and accept them as normal.** When you're facing family changes—whether it's a brother or sister leaving the nest or parents divorcing or a parent remarrying— you're likely to have a lot of different feelings all jumbled up into a confused tangle inside. You may feel sad about losing some part of family togetherness (even as you feel more and more like doing things with your friends), angry that your world is changing because of someone else's choice, scared that no one will love you in quite the same way again, scared that a sibling will change during his or her time away or that if one parent leaves your day-to-day life, he or she will leave you forever or, if you have a parent remarrying into another family with kids, you may be scared that there won't be enough love and attention to go around. Do these describe any of your feelings? They're not so unusual. You have lots and lots of company. Change *can* be sad and scary and make you pretty mad when it isn't something you would have chosen. Just remember that feelings can't be judged. They just happen as they happen. What does matter is what you do about your feelings.

When you're having a lot of different feelings that are making you hurt inside, there are several ways you can express these. You can be angry and sulky around your departing sibling. You can tell your divorcing parents that you hate them and that they're ruining your life. You can do everything you can to make a prospective stepmom or stepdad think twice and run for the hills. Or not. If you choose to express your feelings in a negative way, you'll probably just feel worse. The same is true if you decide to show your family just how upset you are by getting into fights at school, not doing your homework or getting into big trouble on a daily basis.

So what are you supposed to do when you feel so bad? It might help to admit more directly that you're feeling upset, scared, furious or whatever you're feeling. Talk about it. Cry about it with family members or friends or even a favorite teacher, school counselor or professional counselor. When you're able to face your pain and talk about it, you can see, first of all, that you're not alone, and you can survive these changes and re-discover how much you have to look forward to in life.

■ **Don't blame yourself for your parents' divorce.** Young people often do this because they hate feeling so powerless in the midst of such a huge family change. If you think you caused the pending divorce in some way, then maybe you think you can stop it. That's kind of how the thinking goes, even if you're not totally aware of it. The fact is, even if your parents, in their own anger and sadness, say you've driven them to divorce, don't believe it! A strong, loving marriage can survive many family storms and stresses. Your parents are breaking up for their *own* reasons, reasons that you may never understand—or may know all too well. When you realize that this crisis is not your fault, it can be both scary and liberating. It's scary because you realize you can't do anything to change the situation. It's liberating because you're free to love and continue to have warm relationships with both parents, if that's what you choose to do.

■ **Find new ways of building closeness.** This can mean lots of e-mails and, yes, even snail-mail, to your brother or sister now living away from home. It can mean new activities with a parent who is living apart from the family or finding special time to talk with a parent who has become less available to you by returning to work or getting a time-intensive new job or promotion. If you make a decision to stay close, you can do it. Sometimes you may find yourself writing something to a loved one that you'd be embarrassed to say to them in person—and so you grow closer still. When time is more limited with a parent for any reason, you're not as likely to take time together for granted, and time spent together is even more precious.

■ **Give your family changes a fair chance.** A parental divorce hurts—a lot! In fact, a study on divorce by Dr. Paul Dworkin, associate chairman of the Department of Pediatrics at the University of Connecticut School of Medicine, found that, while the first year after a parental divorce is the hardest, with lots of anxiety, sadness, anger, guilt and being scared about the future, some 37 percent of the group studied were still having lots of problems at home or at school five years later. The number of young people having problems 10 years after their parents' divorces rose to 41 percent. Those who did the best had parents who had loving relationships with their children and respectful, considerate relationships with each other, protecting their kids from bitterness and fighting. The time after a divorce is a big adjustment for everyone. But it can, and usually does, get better with time and effort. In the same way, if one or both parents decide to remarry, you may be totally appalled by his or her choice of mate or by the fact that this new mate comes equipped with an instant blended family. Love and acceptance take time to develop. Maybe your new blended family will be a close and reasonably happy one in time. Or maybe it won't. But it makes sense to give everyone a chance. You may or may not come to love each other, but it *is* possible to learn to tolerate each other. It's just easier to live that way instead of being in constant combat. In the meantime, you may find a support group for teens with divorced parents at school or at your local community center. This may be a chance to air all those feelings that you can't express freely (and keep family peace) at home and begin to heal from this major heartbreak.

■ **Discover what positive things your family changes have brought to your life.** When you're feeling sad or scared or so mad you can hardly stand it, it's hard to imagine anything positive could come out of some painful or difficult family changes. But think for a moment. You can't keep these changes from happening or change something that is really someone else's decision. But you can change your own thinking about the situation. We always have a choice. You can think about your parents' divorce and tell yourself that no sane person would ever get married and that you'll never let any person get close enough to you ever again to hurt you so much. Or you can think about how you would like your life to be different and that, as you begin to understand better why your parents couldn't be together any longer, you may vow to work extra hard at making your love relationships work and to learn a little from your parents' painful example.

A positive way of looking at other family changes can help, too. If a brother or sister decides to go to college far away (instead of the local school that everybody just automatically attends), this breaks new ground for you. You might find when your turn comes, that you'll want to go away to school, too, and will have learned a lot from watching your sibling go through the experience first. Or you may decide, with full knowledge of what going away would be like, that your preference is to stay closer to home. And if a parent's increased working hours have meant more responsibility for you, you also have a choice. You can moan and groan and feel burdened by new household chores and responsibilities. Or you can choose to see these new responsibilities as a way to grow to competent adulthood sooner than your friends—who *still* may not have a clue about cooking an edible dinner or doing laundry or shopping for the family. If you are growing up learning all these independent living skills, you'll be at a real advantage when you are on your own.

These are just some ideas. The important thing to remember is that, even in instances where you may have no choice about certain family changes, you *do* have a choice about how you decide to think about the situation and whether it will affect your life in positive as well as negative ways.

Your Growing Independence

Why is it that parents get so embarrassing when they get older? I used to get along great with my mom and be so proud of my dad, but now they both embarrass me all the time. They're always saying or doing or wearing things that just make me want to run and hide from my friends. Why is that? How can I get them to stop embarrassing me? ✳ SUZI C.

I'm always getting into hassles with my parents. Like my mother will just about have a stroke if I leave my schoolbooks in the kitchen instead of taking them to my room. She has this rule about not leaving stuff around in places it doesn't belong. Why does she get so upset when I always move my books to my room after a while? She keeps reminding me and nagging as if I were a 2-year-old! ✳ JOSH L.

Independence is a gradual process that begins when you're a toddler and really picks up speed during puberty and adolescence. You begin doing more and more things for yourself, making many more of your own decisions, until—by your late teens or early to mid-twenties—you're on your own completely.

Growing toward independence isn't easy. If you're like most people, you have a lot of mixed feelings about it. You may want to be on your own and yet need your parents very much sometimes. It can be really confusing—both to you and your parents! There are a number of signs that happen around the time of puberty that show you're starting your real push for independence.

One of the first signs is your changing perception of your parents. When you were a little kid, they were your whole world. You probably thought they were perfect, that they could do no wrong. Now, if you're like many preteens and young teenagers, your parents seem to have trouble doing anything right.

Even though they may have changed a bit, it's more likely that *your* view of them has changed. You're older. You know more. And you realize that your parents—like anyone else—can't possibly be perfect. Maybe it feels very disappointing to you to find that out. Maybe you're afraid that your friends will judge you by your parents' faults, weaknesses and imperfections. It may take a while to feel enough separateness from your parents to realize that your dad's loud Hawaiian shirt or your mother's strange laugh have nothing to do with you.

Some experts feel, too, that many young adolescents *need* to get critical of their parents in order to get ready to leave them. One psychologist remarked to us that some kids, in order to get ready to leave the nest, need to batter the nest up a little, to convince themselves that they're not leaving much of value behind. For some, that's the only way that separation is possible.

Of course, it's also quite possible to grow to independence still feeling close to your parents and realizing every moment how special they are. But as you grow up—whether or not you are critical of your parents—you will begin to see them more and more as human beings with strong and weak points instead of simply as parents.

Another sign that you're beginning your push for independence is your desire for more and more freedom. You may begin to challenge your parents' rules, test their boundaries, want more privileges and, not too surprisingly, have more disagreements with them.

In a very real sense, that's what Josh seems to be expressing. He knows his mother doesn't want stray schoolbooks in the kitchen. Putting them there anyway is his way of testing her rules and trying to show that he is an independent person who can make up his own mind about when the books will end up in his room.

But there's more to it than that. If Josh were truly independent, he might decide to put his books where he could most easily find them for studying: at his desk, in his room. By leaving them in the kitchen, he is inviting nagging from his mother. And that nagging can keep them connected. He complains that his mother's constant reminders are ones she might give to a 2-year-old. But it could be that Josh, even while asserting his growing independence, has moments of wanting to be a little kid and have his mother tell him every move to make.

That's also a normal part of growing into independence. There may be times when you feel very grown up, confident and in control of things. Then you'll have moments, even whole days, when you don't feel grown-up at all. You want to be protected and taken care of by your parents. Then, suddenly, you're wanting to be on your own again! This taking two steps forward and one step back is a way of adjusting to your growing up in your own time and your own way. It isn't always an easy time for you—or your parents.

Your need to become independent may keep you from expressing loving feelings for your parents at times. You may, in fact, think that to feel and express love for them will trap you forever in childhood. But the opposite may be true. The more separate you become, the more you see and understand your parents as people (even when you disagree with them), the deeper your love for them can grow. This usually takes some years to evolve, but it does happen in many families by a young person's late teens or early twenties.

In the meantime, good communication is the key to living with each other's differences. Seeing each other as separate people, listening to and caring about each other, even when you don't agree, is what good communication is all about.

Good communication isn't always easy. It takes time and effort. And it takes a lot of mutual respect. You need to allow each other to make mistakes and have off-days. It's not reasonable to expect your parents to be perfect or to change all their views or tastes to agree with yours or to completely devote their lives to doing what you want to do. At the same time, you have a right to have some time and tastes and dreams of your own.

If you and your parents can begin to accept your growing separateness, if you can agree with joy and disagree with as much gentleness and respect as possible, you're on your way to building a very special new relationship. You may have some difficult times. You may end up having very different lives, thoughts and dreams. But, with love and communication, you can get through the tough times and find new joy in being yourselves and sharing your lives together!

Depression And Grief

I'm not sure what's wrong with me. I get upset a lot and get into fights with my parents and my friends, and now everyone's mad at me. I can't concentrate, and my grades are going down. Sometimes I can't sleep and sometimes I want to sleep all the time. And lots of times I cry for no reason. My mom wants me to go to the doctor, but I'm too scared because what if something is really, really wrong with me? What can I do??? ✳ MEGAN B.

I have a stupid problem. It feels stupid and also horrible. This past year, my brother died from cancer and I miss him a lot. He was only one year older, so we were pretty close. My mom cries all the time. My dad just sits around not saying much or gets mad at me for the smallest thing. I think he wishes I had died instead of Rob. I cry a lot and feel like I'll never be happy again and, worst of all, I'm mad at Rob for dying and changing everything in our family because of that. Is that totally crazy? Is something really wrong with me? ✳ SAM J.

I have a problem I'm embarrassed to ask anyone I know and that is, are you really stupid if you're more upset about your cat dying than about your grandma? The reason I'm asking is that my grandma in Las Vegas died in January. I was sad and all, especially for my dad because she was his mother. But I only saw this grandma a couple of times that I remember, and she wasn't as nice or as interested in me as my other grandma. Mostly, all I remember is that she smoked a lot, she had a gold tooth near the front that showed when she smiled and she once gave me a silver dollar. She was sort of a stranger other than that. My cat Edith Ann died about a month after Grandma Ruby, and I can't stop crying about her. I am so upset! And my dad says I have a real problem if I get more upset about a cat than about my grandma. Is that true? I felt so close to my cat. I'd tell her everything and cuddle her and it was like she was my best friend! Is that normal or not? ✳ COURTNEY Y.

In her letter, Megan is describing very common symptoms of depression. Sam and Courtney are dealing with feelings of grief, having lost loved ones, including dearly loved pets, close to them. Although depression and grief can sometimes look the same, they're different in some ways, too.

Grief is a process that you go through when you experience a loss. This loss may be the loss of a much-loved relative, friend or pet. You can also experience grief when you lose some other aspect of your life that you treasure. For example, you may grieve over the loss of a special relationship if someone you love a lot moves away or doesn't share your feelings of wanting to be close. You may grieve the loss of your friends, your school and your daily routine if your family has to move. You may feel grief if you lose a treasured goal—if, for example, a physical injury cuts short your dreams for a career in ballet or of being an Olympic gymnast.

We say that grief is a process because it isn't just one feeling, but a lot of different feelings. At first, you might feel numb, then denial or disbelief (as in, "No, this can't really be happening!" or "This is not happening!").

Then you might feel a lot of anger. This could be like the anger that Sam describes in his letter—anger at a person who died for leaving you or changing your life. As selfish or strange as it may feel, this is a normal part of the grief process. You might feel anger at your parents if their choice or need to move from your former home meant leaving behind people you love or your whole life as you've known it. You may feel anger at yourself or at your teacher or coach if you've suffered a dream-ending physical injury.

You might also feel a lot of guilt for a time, telling yourself that if you had just spent more time with the person, or shown your love a little more, or been more careful in doing warm-ups, this loss would not have happened.

After this, you may feel bereavement, overwhelming sadness about losing someone you loved so much—whether that was a person or a companion animal or a dream or goal for the future.

After all this, the numbness, denial, anger, guilt and tears, comes acceptance. That doesn't mean that you say it's O.K. or forget about the person or never feel sad again. It simply means that this loss becomes a part of your life without stopping you from living your normal, everyday life. Maybe you'll always feel a bit sad inside, always missing your lost loved one. But you realize that you need to go on with your life while keeping warm memories of that person to comfort you in sad moments.

How can you get through this grief process?

■ **Let your feelings happen.** Each person has his or her own way of grieving. So do you. If you feel like crying, cry. If you feel like talking with someone close to you, do. If you feel like saying something in a private moment to the person you have lost or writing about your feelings in a journal, that's O.K., too. Crying and showing your pain isn't a sign of weakness. Facing painful feelings takes courage, and tears can be healing.

■ **Don't judge your reactions to a loss.** Others might tell you that you *should* feel more upset about losing a person than a pet or a relative than a friend. But that isn't how it always is in real life. A much-loved pet you've had for years may be much closer to you in spirit than a grandparent who lives far away and whom you see only occasionally. The loss of the pet will have a much greater impact on your daily life, and so it's not so surprising if, like Courtney, you find yourself crying more about the death of a pet than that of a distant relative. In the same way, the death of a friend or classmate can be upsetting in a whole different way than the loss of an elderly relative whose death was not unexpected. When a friend dies, you're not only losing that friend, but also your sense of safety and youthful immortality. You know now, for sure, that bad things can happen to good people, no matter how young or promising they may have been. What's important is to just let your feelings happen. If you're not as upset as your parent about the death of a grandparent, here's a chance to be extra supportive and kind to your grieving parent. If you feel overwhelming sadness about the death of a pet or of a friend, this just as normal as crying over the loss of a much-loved relative.

■ **Talk to others about how you feel.** This might mean talking about your feelings or talking about the person or pet you lost. Think about the people in your life who might listen. Think about joining a grief group for teens who have experienced similar losses. Sometimes it can be a relief to know other people are experiencing a lot of what you're feeling. You don't feel quite so strange—or alone.

■ **Realize that the grief process isn't a predictable thing.** Some days you may feel pretty normal and then, that night or the next day, you can't stop crying. That just happens. Having a day when you're fairly happy and enjoying your life doesn't mean that you didn't love the person you lost. And experiencing another wave of grief when you were just starting to feel a little bit yourself again doesn't mean you've gone totally crazy. That's how grief is. It comes and goes and sometimes catches you by surprise. You'll grow toward acceptance in your own way and in your own time. In the meantime, enjoy your good days. Learning to laugh and to experience the joys of life fully in between your moments of pain can help you heal.

Depression, unlike grief, may or may not be due to a specific event in your life. It's true that you can feel depressed when your best friend won't speak to you or when you don't make a team or when you worked really hard to get a "B" in math and your parents are still disappointed because it's not an "A." But, like Megan, you can also be depressed for no specific reason. Depression can be a complex mix of social, psychological and/or physical factors. Some people may always feel a little depressed. Some get very depressed for a certain time and then are O.K.

The symptoms of depression aren't always obvious. True, some depressed people look sad. But others, particularly teens, get very irritable and angry. Some get into fights at school or say mean things to their friends. Some other signs of depression are:

■ Loss of interest or enjoyment in things you've always liked to do before

■ A change in eating habits—like eating more than usual and gaining weight or feeling too upset to eat at all

■ Having trouble getting to sleep at night or feeling like you want to sleep all the time

■ Feeling jumpy or restless or like you're living in slow motion

■ Feeling tired all the time

■ Feeling worthless or hopeless just about every day

■ Having trouble remembering stuff that's usually easy to recall or being unable to concentrate

■ Feeling like giving up or even dying

How can you deal with depression?

1. *Get moving!* Exercise can help a lot. Go for a walk. Dance to upbeat music. Hit a tennis ball against the wall—or pursue a sport you've enjoyed in the past. Getting out and getting active not only

helps distract you and change the pace of your life, but also it can help the flow of beneficial hormones called *endorphins* throughout your body. These endorphins give you a sensation of well-being. (If you've ever heard people talk about a "runner's high," they're talking about the action of endorphins in a person's body after a vigorous run or other exercise.)

2. *Look for positive, not negative, ways to feel better.* Like what? Talk with a friend or with your parents. Write in your journal or diary. Pound pillows if you're feeling angry and frustrated. Cry if that's what you feel like doing. Do something good for yourself or for someone else, even if that's the last thing you really feel like doing. Things to avoid: alcohol or drugs. Some teens try these to keep from feeling pain, but these can bring you down even more. They are a problem, not a solution!

3. *Act as if you weren't depressed and see if you don't start feeling better.* Sometimes people who are depressed get into a negative mood that's hard to shake because they start to act depressed. They hide in their rooms, refuse to get together with friends or do anything fun and so they get even more depressed. Sometimes you can begin to feel better by breaking this pattern of feeling bad. Ask yourself what you would do right now if you weren't depressed— and then *do* it. Call a friend. Say "Yes" to a suggestion to go to a movie or for a walk in the park or to the mall. When you get up and out into the world, things can start to look a little brighter.

4. *Give yourself something to look forward to every day.* No matter how small it is, having a reason to look forward to tomorrow can do a lot to help lift your depression today.

5. *If nothing is helping, talk with your parents about getting professional help.* A good place to start might be your regular doctor. It's a good idea to get checked out to make sure that nothing physical is the matter. Some illnesses, like mononucleosis, can make

people feel depressed and tired. If there is no special physical reason for your down mood, your doctor might suggest that you see a counselor, psychologist or psychotherapist. All of these titles are used to describe people who will listen to you and then help you find ways to help yourself. They're not going to try to change your total personality or make you feel weird or convince you and those around you that you're totally crazy. Many people never end up getting professional help because they manage to pull themselves out of depression or have family or friends they can talk with and feel better. But if, despite your best efforts and those of your family and friends, you're still feeling hopeless, a professional can help you and maybe even your whole family (if that's what you choose) deal with feelings that are hard for you and those close to you to understand. Some people even need medication for a time so that their depression will lift enough so that they can begin to help themselves.

6. *If you feel like dying or like hurting yourself in any way, tell your parents or another trusted adult. And remember that as long as there is life, there is hope.* Many people who say they want to die simply want to live differently. Seek help in beginning to live differently. If you're desperate and feel there's no one in your life to talk with, pick up the phone and ask the operator for the number of the local Suicide Prevention Hotline. Or you can call the Boys Town National Hot Line (they help girls as well as boys): 1-800-448-3000. You will find someone on the other end who will listen and tell you where to get help in your area. There *is* help, no matter how hopeless or alone you may be feeling.

Just remember that no matter how bad you feel, there is help and there is hope. Whatever has happened—whether you lost someone special in your life or your best pet ever or if you feel worthless and pessimistic about your life ever getting any better—time and people who care can help.

New Loves In Your Life

Is it normal for a 12-year-old boy (that's me) to be in love with a neighbor-lady who's 24 and married? She's real nice to me and likes to hear all about my computer games and stuff. I think she's beautiful, and I think I love her. Is it possible that she could love me, too? Sometimes I feel real shy because I had a dream about her being naked once and got really turned on. I feel funny about that because she's a very nice lady and, like I said, she's married. ✳ ANDY W.

Please don't use my name because this is very embarrassing. What I want to know is, do normal people love and admire and want to be with someone who's the same sex? I really love my best girlfriend and there's this English teacher at school I admire so much, I think of her all the time. I think she's just perfect. What's the matter with me? Does this mean I'm gay? ✳ WONDERING

I'm Toby Maguire's biggest fan ever, and I think of him all the time. It's like I'm in love with him and have daydreams about him even though we've never met. My dad says this is silly and immature. My older brother says I'm just plain crazy. Am I?
✳ WONDERING IN WASHINGTON

Is it possible for two people to love each other before they're really teenagers? I'm 11 and have a boyfriend, Rick, who just turned 12. We love each other a lot, but no one takes it seriously. They keep laughing about "puppy love." But I've never felt this way about anyone before. What's the difference between puppy love and real love? I KNOW what we feel is real love! ✳ JESSICA A.

As your independence grows, you may begin to feel a need to be close to people outside your family. You may find new people to love and admire. This love can take many forms.

You may find yourself getting crushes on adults you know—teachers or neighbors or friends of the family. Or you may feel overwhelming love for a performer you've never met but whose music or acting has touched your emotions and inspired your fantasies in a special way.

Having crushes or loving someone from afar is a normal, even necessary, part of growing up. Why? Because you're having a lot of new feelings and needs right now.

First, you're beginning to grow away from your parents little by little and want to feel quite separate from them a lot of the time. But you still need people to listen and to help you sort things out. Your friends probably do this a lot. But they have their own growing up tasks and problems. Sometimes they're so caught up in their own feelings and experiences, they can't listen to you at the moment. That's when it's nice to have an older friend to turn to.

Second, you're beginning to have new feelings and desires. You may feel attracted to the opposite sex in a new way. You might even imagine yourself in romantic or sexual scenes with someone. A lot of people your age have such thoughts and feelings. These just happen and can't be called good or bad—just normal. It's what you *do* that matters. It's quite likely that you aren't ready to do much, if anything, about these new feelings. Having fantasies about people you like or feeling attracted to someone you know isn't available, whether this is an older person, married or unmarried, or a celebrity, is a way to get used to your new feelings without really having to do anything about them.

Loving, *nonexploitive* friendships with older people can help you a lot. Nonexploitive means that the older person doesn't expect anything unusual, including sexual involvement, from you. It means that this older friend is most interested in helping you feel good about yourself.

Crushes on older people—whether these are people you actually know or celebrities—can also help you discover important qualities in yourself and ways in which you want to grow. Maybe you admire a same-sex teacher because, deep down, you really want to have some of the same admirable qualities he or she has. It's a normal way of finding new ways to be and to grow.

The same is true when you love and admire a close friend. You can see an admirable same-sex person as an important role model, someone to be like in ways you choose. It does *not* usually mean you're gay. Gays, or homosexuals, are people who as *adults* find that they love primarily or exclusively those of the same sex.

Even though right now you may have only dreams and fantasies of turning a faraway celebrity love or a crush on an older friend into reality, it's important to remember that loving someone in your heart, from afar, is just as real in its own way as loving a boyfriend or girlfriend later on. The difference is that now you can experience this love in a way that allows you to have these warm feelings without the risks of being taken advantage of or getting physically involved with someone before you're ready. Experimenting with love in your heart and your imagination is a very important and special part of growing up!

So is loving a first boyfriend or girlfriend. It's possible to love someone of the same general age and of the opposite sex very much when you're young. A lot of older people may smile and say it's just puppy love. What some mean by this is that it's love that can't last because you and the other person are changing so much and are too inexperienced with love and life to make a total commitment. What others mean is that young love has an innocent, playful quality to it that is wonderfully unique. But don't let these opinions confuse your feelings. You *can* be in love at a young age. Young love *is* real.

Love has no age limits. But, as you grow and change emotionally, the character of your love may change. You tend to love in different ways as you grow to know yourself better and to feel more secure in who you are. Your way of loving may grow and change as you become more independent. But love at any age, in any form, whether it lasts for a lifetime or for only a short but memorable time, is a wonderful part of life.

Getting To Know The Real You

Sometimes I just can't figure myself out! There are times when I feel like a little kid and cry when I think about someday moving away from home. Then there are times when I dream about what my life will be like when I have my own place and a job and a car and I get really excited and can hardly wait! And I'm not sure who I really am, what my personality is like or what I really want out of life. Does this make any sense? ✳ MEGAN C.

Megan expresses the feelings of many young people in transition. Your past and your future may be much on your mind as you cope with the present.

The person you're growing to be may seem very new and grown-up in some ways, yet very familiar in other ways. You will always carry some of the child you once were inside. It's quite common, at this point in your life, to feel a bit sad over the loss of your childhood. But you don't have to leave everything behind just because you're growing up! You don't have to give up the parts of your child-self that you like and value. You can always be curious or playful or get excited over small things. That can bring a lot of joy and fun to your life as an adult.

When you're not quite sure who you are or how to be, though, you find that your feelings are tender and easily hurt. You're far from alone. That's why it's so important to be gentle, not only with yourself, but also with your friends and classmates during this time of change.

Being kind to yourself and others instead of being critical, giving yourself and others the room to make mistakes (which can help you learn a lot about yourself) can help you to grow up feeling good about yourself and the world around you.

This time in between childhood and adulthood, when you're trying to find out who you are, is confusing. It's normal to wonder how you fit into the world and who you really are.

Self-discovery is something people pursue for a lifetime. You can't be expected to figure it all out today, tomorrow or by next year. But you can start to know yourself better by deciding—maybe even writing it all down in a diary or journal—what you think and believe about everyday things or unusual events. Who are the people you love most—and what makes them so special to you? What are the things you like most to do? If you could plan a perfect day for yourself, what would it be like? What do you like most about yourself so far? Least?

The best part of growing up is becoming aware of your likes and dislikes, your unique talents and abilities, your special interests and your dreams, and giving yourself the freedom just to be yourself—whether it is enjoying the child you've been or the young adult you're growing to be!

9

Coping with the Common Problems of Puberty

What are growing pains? Why do they happen? I have them and it scares me. Will they interfere with any growing? When will they go away? ✻ AMY Y.

I'm 12 and have a pain in my hip and knee and have started limping. My mom wants me to go to the doctor but I don't want to because he'll nag me about my weight again. Last time I went he said I needed to lose 40 pounds! What do I have and what is the doctor likely to do about it? Does it have anything to do with being over-weight? ✻ DON H.

I'm 10 years old and love ballet! I take three dance classes a week. But I've been having some swelling around my knee and it hurts! If I go to the doctor, I know she'll say I have to stop dancing and I don't want to do that. What's the matter with my knee? Could I just do something at home to help it instead of going to the doctor? ✻ MELISSA O.

Ll these letters describe some of the common problems young
people can face during puberty.

If you're like most people, your first reaction to an unusual
pain or occurrence is fear that something might be seriously wrong.
Then you get worried about it interfering with important activities you
enjoy. You might be too scared or embarrassed to mention your symptoms to anyone. So you keep it all secret or try to ignore it as much as
you can. But keeping secrets like this can hurt you even more. It's
important to mention your pain or symptoms to your parents and your
doctor. Help is available for all the common problems of puberty.

In some cases, the sooner you get help the less pain this problem
will cause you *and* the less likely it is to interfere with your active life.
Also, the less you worry and wonder and the more you know and
understand about your body, the better you'll feel!

Here are the facts about some of the most common problems preteens and young teenagers have.

Growing Pains

*I'm 11 years old and have pains in my legs, especially at night. My
mom took me to our doctor and after examining me, he said that nothing serious was wrong, that I just had growing pains. What are growing
pains? What can I do about them? My parents and doctor don't seem
to think they matter much, but my legs HURT!!* ✼ SHANNON S.

Growing pains are quite common during periods of rapid growth.
Although they occur most frequently between the ages of 5 and 13,
they reach a peak in girls at about age 10 or 11 and in boys when they
are about 13.

What are the symptoms? You'll have pain that comes and goes in the muscles of your legs and thighs. The most common places to feel these pains are behind your knee and in the front of your thighs and along your shins. Some young people also feel pains in their arms, back, groin or shoulders, but these are less common. Growing pains often happen late in the day or at night. They usually don't keep you from getting around. You're not likely to notice any swelling in your legs. But your legs *do* hurt!

It isn't really known why growing pains happen, but you're most likely to have them when you're growing fast. If you have these pains, tell your parents and check with your doctor. Growing pains are not harmful, will not interfere with your growth and do not need medical treatment. However, it's important for your doctor to make sure that these are, in fact, growing pains and not symptoms of other conditions that do need medical treatment.

Growing pains go away in time, as your growth slows down. In the meantime, you can ease your pain by gently massaging the areas that are hurting, putting a heating pad on the painful spots and taking an aspirin or aspirin-substitute. (It's important to be aware that Reye's syndrome, a rare but serious disease, has been linked with aspirin use in children during viral infections such as flu or chicken pox. If you have either condition or are uncertain about what may be causing your pain, check with your parents and your doctor before taking aspirin.)

Gynecomastia

I'm getting breasts and I'm a boy. There is swelling under my nipples and they're sore to touch. What's the matter with me??? I'm too embarrassed to tell anyone I know, so please tell me what to do about this! ✳ RYAN P.

Gynecomastia is a very common, temporary enlargement of the breasts that happens to a lot of growing boys (about 20 percent of 10-year-olds and 64 percent of 14-year-olds). It seems to be caused by hormonal increases and, perhaps, a slight hormonal imbalance that often can occur during early puberty.

There are some boys who get gynecomastia as the result of drug use (especially marijuana) or as part of an illness. Others, who are quite overweight, often have breasts somewhat enlarged with fat tissue. But most boys have this temporary breast tenderness and enlargement as a part of the hormonal changes of puberty.

What are the signs of gynecomastia? You may get a nodule underneath the areola in one or both breasts. In some instances, this nodule, an area of firm swelling, will extend beyond the areola. Other boys get overall breast enlargement that resembles stage three of female breast development. In this last instance, the breasts will feel somewhat like female breasts. When there is only a nodule, however, the breasts will be firm and tender to the touch.

It's a good idea to check with your doctor to make sure that you do have gynecomastia. Most of the time, gynecomastia goes away within a year to 18 months, so your doctor is most likely to reassure you that you are normal and tell you that this is a temporary condition. Surgery is not usually recommended for this condition. Only in *very* rare instances when the breasts are extremely large and the gynecomastia shows no sign of going away within the expected time frame will surgery be performed to reduce the size of the breasts. However, this is very rarely necessary.

If you're getting teased about it, remember that gynecomastia *is* temporary and it doesn't mean that you're turning into a woman or that you're not as masculine as everyone else.

Menstrual Problems

IRREGULARITY

I had my first period seven months ago. I had one period and then I didn't have another one for three months. The next one I had was heavy and then I didn't have another one for two more months. Is all of this normal? ✳ KATIE F.

As we discussed in Chapter Three, it is quite common to have irregular periods in the first year or so after you begin to menstruate.

Why does this happen? Your hormonal levels are still changing a lot, and your own individual timing of your periods may not be set quite yet. It's very common to have a pattern like Katie's: getting a heavy period and then none at all for several months.

You can expect to get regular monthly menstrual periods within two years after you begin menstruating or by age 18. Normal cycles can vary a lot in length. For example, some women menstruate every four weeks (or 28 days). Others have their periods every three-and-a-half weeks and still others menstruate every five weeks. Being regular means establishing a cycle that's consistent and normal for *you!*

Things like emotional stress or traveling (and jet lag) can also cause your periods to become temporarily irregular. However, if these are not factors and if you've been menstruating for two years or more and only then become irregular, this may be a sign of a physical problem requiring your doctor's examination and advice.

PREMENSTRUAL SYMPTOMS

I sometimes gain weight just before my period and have headaches. Why does this happen? Is this premenstrual syndrome? How do I get rid of it? ✳ ERIN O.

Weight gain, headaches, fatigue and tender breasts are some symptoms women can get before their periods. Most women just get a symptom or two from time to time. Those who have premenstrual syndrome (PMS), on the other hand, have symptoms so regular and severe that these interfere with their normal life at school and at home.

Why do such symptoms occur? They're usually due to water retention in your body. As your hormonal level changes (estrogen decreases and progesterone increases) just before your menstrual period, your kidneys filter less water and salt from your body. This excess water is then retained in your body tissues, causing breast soreness or headaches or that overall bloated feeling.

How can you help avoid these symptoms?

■ **Cut down your salt intake in general, but especially in the week before your period is due.** This means cutting out or cutting down on salty foods such as soft drinks (they're sweet but have a lot of hidden salt in them), hot dogs, potato chips and other snack foods, lunch meats, bacon, sausage, ham and canned foods.

■ **Eliminate caffeine.** If you tend to get sore breasts before your period, cutting out caffeine—which is found in cola drinks, hot chocolate, coffee and tea—can help.

■ **Eat smaller but more frequent meals of protein and complex carbohydrates.** Have a small meal every three hours in the week before your period. Eat fresh fruit, eggs, rice, cheese, peanuts, yogurt and whole wheat bread. Bananas, tomatoes and apricots, which contain potassium, can help relieve symptoms such as headaches and water retention. Also, don't go for long periods without food. (This is one of the most common causes of premenstrual headaches, especially in girls who are dieting.)

■ **Relax as much as you can.** Emotional stress can make premenstrual symptoms worse. If you're tense, take a warm bath or listen to music you especially like. Close your eyes and breathe deeply, telling your body to relax. Cuddle your pet. Take a nap or go to bed a little early.

■ **Take vitamins.** Some medical experts believe that vitamin B_6 can help alleviate or prevent premenstrual symptoms. Some believe, too, that taking two or three calcium supplements (up to 1,000 mgs.) daily in the 10 days before menstruation may help alleviate PMS symptoms.

■ **Exercise.** Being physically active can ease stress and can help prevent the depression and irritability some women feel during premenstrual days. Do whatever exercise you enjoy. Or, if you don't really like or feel up to any particular form of exercise, take a walk. Walk your dog. Walk instead of asking for a ride to school or to your friend's house. Or take a brisk stroll by yourself around the neighborhood. Amazing, but true: Walking (or some other form of exercise) can be a real energy booster when you're feeling tired, depressed or otherwise not at your best.

If your symptoms persist or are very severe, see your doctor. There are prescription medicines that can help if you actually have premenstrual syndrome. Some doctors treat the problem with natural estrogen and/or progesterone. Some physicians will give young women with PMS who are old enough to need a reliable method of birth control the new triphasic oral contraceptives that can alleviate PMS symptoms as well.

MENSTRUAL CRAMPS

Are cramps really just all in your head? That's what my friend Sara says. But I think I have a good attitude about menstruation and my body and I STILL get cramps sometimes! Why does this happen and what can I do? ✳ BETH C.

Menstrual cramps are *not* all in your head! They're real and are caused by a possible overproduction of substances known as prostaglandins. These cause the uterus to contract, which, in turn, can cause cramps.

If you have mild cramps, you might try:

■ **Aspirin.** Aspirin contains anti-prostaglandins as well as pain relievers. Bufferin and Advil also contain anti-prostaglandins.

Tylenol does not have these substances. (See page 166 concerning aspirin and Reye's syndrome.)

■ **Heat in moderate amounts.** Rest for a while with a warm heating pad or take a warm bath.

■ **Exercise.** A recent study shows that some 70 percent of teens who had suffered from cramps but who had then begun to exercise daily had far less menstrual pain within only a few months. The daily exercise you choose doesn't have to be a major sport. Swimming or taking a brisk walk or fast dancing to your favorite music may be just what your body needs. Not that long ago, women used to be advised to avoid exercise during menstruation, but now we know that it can actually help relieve cramps.

If your cramps are really severe, help is available. See your doctor. He or she will want to examine you to make sure that you have no other medical condition that could be causing your pain. Then your doctor may prescribe a special prostaglandin-inhibiting drug like Motrin or Ponstel in small doses for a few days each month to help alleviate your cramps.

If your cramps persist, your doctor may prescribe estrogen/progesterone combination pills, usually called birth control pills, but also these are useful in regulating your menstrual cycle and decreasing both your cramps and the number of days you have your period.

As a last resort, your doctor might prescribe prescription painkillers. This is usually only done if you're allergic to aspirin and other anti-prostaglandins and also can't take hormone pills.

Osgood-Schlatter Disease

I'm on the varsity basketball team this year—which is great. But what's not so great is that I'm having a lot of pain in my left knee. My doctor told me this means I have some sort of disease and I shouldn't play basketball. Is this true? What can I do so I can still play? I've really worked hard to get on the team! ❅ EVAN W.

Osgood-Schlatter Disease is quite common among active adolescents. It occurs more frequently in males than females. It's most likely to afflict those who are in the period of rapid growth: Girls are most likely to have it around the age of 10 or 11 and boys around the age of 12 or 13.

This disorder happens when the anterior upper portion of the lower leg (the shin bone) is not yet fully calcified as it will be in adulthood. During the rapid growth time of puberty, the muscle pulls against the soft cartilage of this not-yet-hardened bone. This pulling and muscle strain causes pain and swelling around this part of the leg. If you have such symptoms, check with your doctor.

The reassuring thing is that Osgood-Schlatter Disease will go away in time. However, your doctor may suggest that you stay away from vigorous sports or exercises involving knee-bending for a certain amount of time. Some young people find that resting for two to four weeks will help improve the condition enough to allow them to return to their normal activities. In some instances, your doctor may suggest a longer rest—from several months to as long as a year. During this time, you can still be active but need to limit yourself to sports that don't put extra stress on your knees (e.g., swimming).

If you have an unusually severe case of Osgood-Schlatter Disease, you may need a cast for a short time to help your knee(s) heal, but usually a brief period of rest is enough.

It can be frustrating to stay away from dance class or team practice for several weeks (or even months), but it may help to remember that, once your knees are healed, you'll be able to be as active as ever!

Scoliosis

Our school nurse was looking at our backs yesterday. She said I have a curve in my back called scoliosis. I'm supposed to go to a doctor about it tomorrow. I'm really scared. Will I have to have an operation or something? Will I grow out of it? I'm 10 years old. Help! ✻ TARA L.

Scoliosis, a condition in which your spine curves to one side instead of growing straight, is a common and correctable condition. (See Fig. 9-1.) It's most common in the growing years between 10 and 16. Girls are much more likely to get it than boys. In all, about 10 percent of young people have it to some degree. Especially if it is caught and treated early, scoliosis is correctable and will not cause any deformities in later life. In earlier times, those with this condition became hunchbacks and had other medical problems as they got older. These days, that doesn't have to happen.

What are the symptoms of scoliosis? The earliest symptoms include uneven shoulders and/or hips and prominent shoulder blades. Also, your parents or school nurse or doctor may be able to see an S-shaped curve to your spine as you bend over. In fact, school nurses, in regular exams, spot many cases of scoliosis. If your school nurse tells you that you need to see a doctor about this spinal curvature, you and your parents should do so promptly.

No matter who spots your symptoms, you should see a doctor right away to find out how severe your spine curvature is. Your treatment will depend on how mild or severe the curvature happens to be.

If, for example, you have a mild (less than 20 percent) curvature, you may need no treatment at all. The doctor will prescribe some simple exercises and then will probably want you to check back regularly so that he or she can make sure your curvature is not increasing.

If your curvature is more severe, you may need to wear a device

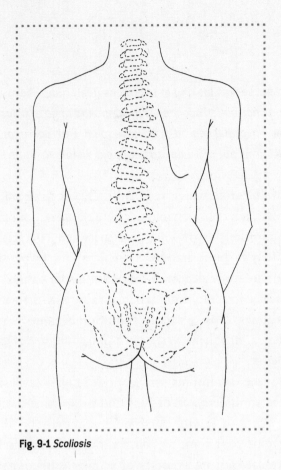

Fig. 9-1 *Scoliosis*

called the Milwaukee brace for a period of time as well as do special exercises. This brace may look pretty cumbersome, but it doesn't have to interfere with your life. One sports-minded young teen we know even continued to play tennis and to run with her brace on! This brace can really help move your spine back into a normal position.

There is a new treatment for scoliosis that is now being tested at fifty medical centers across the United States. This is a painless treatment that uses electrical stimulation of the back muscles during sleep. So far, there is a reported 80 to 90 percent success rate in stopping the spinal curvature among patients who had the treatment every night. These treatments, which could become generally available if the tests continue to go well, could free many teens with scoliosis from having to wear braces at all.

Surgery is performed only rarely, when the spinal curvature is really severe. This surgery involves implanting an adjustable rod to help straighten the spine. Then the teen would also have to have a body cast during recovery from the surgery. But relatively few young people with scoliosis have to have surgery and casting.

It's important to remember that the sooner your scoliosis is detected and treated, the less treatment you'll need! Also, whatever treatment your doctor says is necessary now will benefit you all your life!

Slipped Capital Femoral Epiphysis

> ***I have this pain in my hip and my hip bone has also started clicking! It's so bad I limp a lot. This is scary and embarrassing, too, because I'm overweight and kids make fun of me anyway, but it gets worse when I walk funny. My mother wants to take me to the doctor, but I'm scared to go. What's the matter with me?*** ✻ BRYANT A.

The condition that Bryant is describing is called slipped capital femoral epiphysis. This occurs when the thigh bone (the femur) slips out of place where it connects to the hip.

This usually happens either just before or during a period of rapid growth, between the ages of 10 and 13 in girls and 12 to 15 in boys. Boys are more than twice as likely as girls to have this condition. Of the young people who have slipped capital femoral epiphysis, some 88 percent are very overweight. It is thought that the increased weight that naturally comes with puberty, added to the extra weight an obese young person carries already, may cause this slippage. It happens, experts say, because of too much stress on bones that have not matured enough to carry such weight. (About 70 percent of those with this condition have a bone age that is slightly below their actual chronological age.)

The symptoms of slipped capital femoral epiphysis are pain in your hip or groin, a click in your hip and, quite possibly, a limp. A minority of patients also have some thigh and knee pain. Especially if you're limping, you need to see a doctor promptly.

This condition isn't something that will simply go away. If an examination and x-rays show that you do have slipped capital femoral epiphysis, your doctor will probably refer you to an orthopedic surgeon. Surgery to put the bones back in place and hold them there with tiny wires is the only form of treatment that's totally reliable. Without surgery, damage to the hip could result in a permanent limp.

Surgery may sound scary, but the earlier it is done, the better and more complete your recovery will be.

Backpack Stress And Sports Overload

I really love gymnastics. I've been training since I was 4 and now I'm nearly 12. I keep getting injuries like knee sprains and a stress fracture in my foot. My parents want me to quit but I can't stand the thought. What can I do? ✳ BRONWYN G.

I'm having a lot of back and neck pain and I don't know why. My doctor said it could be because my school backpack is too heavy and that I should get one with wheels but everyone at school would laugh at me if I did that. That is so uncool I can't even think about it! Could it really be my backpack causing a problem, and what can I do? ✳ JASON J.

When your body is in its rapid growth period during the pre-teens and early teens, it's especially important to guard against overtraining and putting too much stress on your back.

That said, we know that some forms of dance and some sports require intensive training during these growing years. Ballet and competitive sports like gymnastics and figure skating require long years of training and practice. But whether you're an aspiring Olympian or ballerina or simply a very active, sports-minded person, common sense is your best defense.

If you notice persistent pain, have a doctor check it out. If he or she says you need to take it easy for a while, do it! It's better to rest and let an injury heal during these growing years than to keep going and risk further damage, even if you're under pressure to work through the injury and pain. It could mean the difference between an injury that ends your dreams and one that interrupts your training or takes you out of competition for a short time.

If you've been noticing a lot of neck and back pain and you lug a heavy backpack to and from school, you might want to make a few changes. The fact is, a heavy backpack can cause back problems during the years of rapid growth between the ages of 10 and 16. A study at the Medical College of Georgia assessed how much force heavy backpacks put on young people ages 10 to 13 as they stepped from a platform onto a high step and back again. The heavier the backpack, the greater force the young people exerted to step up and the greater impact their bodies, mostly their backs, absorbed when they stepped down. These forces put abnormal stresses on the spine and the neck.

Some suggestions to keep your back and neck healthy and trouble-free:

■ **Weigh your backpack and figure out the safest weight to carry.** You shouldn't carry a backpack heavier than 15 percent of your body weight.

■ **Use rolling backpacks when possible.** Even if they've been dorky at your school, they're used more and more. You might even become a trendsetter. Even though backpacks with wheels are better for your back, it's important to use common sense. Don't pack more than you really need . . . because you *still* have to lift them when you're getting out of the bus or car. Be very careful.

- **Carry a backpack properly.** That means using both shoulder straps as well as the additional strap at the waist if your bag has one. Don't try to be macho and swing a heavy bookbag with one hand. It could prove to be a painful mistake.

Tight Foreskin

I read somewhere that if you aren't circumcised you're supposed to pull back your foreskin so you can wash yourself. The problem is, I can't just pull it back because it won't move. It just stays there. What should I do? I'm afraid to tell my doctor because he might say I have to be circumcised and I've heard that's really painful! ✻ JEREMY Y.

Pulling back, or retracting, the foreskin to wash the head of the penis is necessary for good hygiene in the uncircumcised male. If you have a tight foreskin like Jeremy's, check with your doctor. This is a problem that can be corrected fairly easily—and circumcision may not be necessary. A physician, quite often a urologist, will be able to loosen the foreskin, making it retractable.

Frequently, a tight foreskin develops because of poor hygiene; it has not been pulled back often enough to clean the head of the penis thoroughly. Daily retraction and washing are good preventive measures.

Undescended Testicle

I have an unusual problem: I can feel only one testicle. I thought there were supposed to be two. Will I grow another one when I'm older? I'm 13 already and fairly mature. How long should I wait to see if one

grows? I'm too embarrassed to go to a doctor about it. Does having only one ball mean I won't ever be able to have sex or have children?
✲ ALLEN H.

It's possible that Allen has an undescended testicle. Before birth, both testicles are in the baby's abdomen. By birth, however, the testicles have usually descended into the scrotum in most boys. In other cases, the testicle will descend on its own or with medical help sometime between birth and puberty. By puberty, only about 1 boy in 500 will have a testicle still undescended.

If, like Allen, you think you may have an undescended testicle, tell your parents and ask them to take you to a competent doctor for a thorough examination. This may seem very embarrassing, but it's important to your health that you find out for sure.

Why? Because if a testicle is undescended at puberty or beyond, it is particularly vulnerable to developing cancer during the young adult years.

A thorough exam is necessary to determine if your testicle is, in fact, undescended. It isn't as easy to tell as you might think. Some boys have testicles that move up to the groin area and then back to the scrotum from time to time. If you feel that you have such a testicle (called a "floating" testicle), this still needs to be brought to your doctor's attention.

If your testicle is undescended, your physician may recommend that you see a urologist—a medical specialist—who will do a further evaluation and, perhaps, perform surgery to remove the undescended (and usually underdeveloped) testicle.

Even if you do have to have surgery and/or have only one testicle, you are still an entirely normal male. You will be able to have sex and have children just as easily as anyone else. You can manage very well in all ways with only one testicle. However, if you feel embarrassed about perhaps looking a bit different, ask your doctor about a Sialastic testicle implant. This is a special material made the size of a testicle that can fit into the scrotum, making it look as if you have two testicles.

Testicular Torsion

A cousin of a friend of mine had something called testicular torsion and it sounded very serious. Is this very common? How do you know if you have it? ✱ DANIEL S.

Testicular torsion isn't exactly common, but when it happens, immediate treatment is necessary, so it makes sense to learn about it so you know enough to seek help fast!

Testicular torsion happens when a testicle twists around its blood supply cord, trapping blood in the testicle and causing it to swell massively and causing pain in the groin. This condition can come on suddenly, and its main symptom is pain in the groin and, possibly, nausea and vomiting.

How does it happen?

The testicles are quite mobile, moving closer or farther away from the body to maintain a constant temperature so that sperm can develop. Sometimes, in this movement, a testicle can get twisted.

This twisting also can happen during strenuous activity or even during sleep.

If you feel pain in your groin, seek medical help immediately. It may turn out to be due to something else like a sports injury or a hernia or swollen glands. But if you do have testicular torsion, you only have a short time to get help in order to save the affected testicle, which, cut off from its blood supply, can die within four to eight hours.

How is testicular torsion treated?

It is treated through relatively simple surgery. The testicle is untwisted and then fixed into place with a few stitches to keep it from getting twisted again. If you have been able to get medical help soon enough to avoid any additional damage to the testicle, it should be fine and be able to function normally. If you don't get prompt medical attention, the testicle will die, eventually shriveling to the size of a marble and becoming useless. In rare but tragic cases, some people have torsion in both testicles, often at different times, and were not treated in time to have either testicle saved. If one testicle has died but the other is not affected, the surgeon will remove the damaged testicle and then surgically anchor the surviving testicle so it will not be in danger of twisting in the future.

Vaginal Infections

How can you tell if a discharge is normal or if it is the sign of a problem? I have this clear discharge that is supposed to be normal when you're fairly mature (I'm 12 and had my first menstrual period four months ago). But the last week or so I've had this discharge that makes me all red and sore down there and I'm thinking it isn't normal. What's wrong with me? I know it can't be something like VD because I don't even have a boyfriend and I always use toilet seat covers when I use a public bathroom. So what could it be?

✳ JULIE S.

Vaginal infections usually have one major symptom: a discharge that is different in one of several ways from a girl's normal clear-to-whitish discharge. You may have a vaginal infection if you have a discharge that is irritating to your genital area, has a foul odor, causes itching and is a different color from your normal discharge.

The following chart will show the most common vaginal infections and what to do about them.

How can you prevent vaginal infections? The best way is to have a good hygiene routine:

Most Common Vaginal Infections

Infection	Cause	Symptoms	Treatment
Bacterial vaginosis	Vulnerable during times of stress or while taking antibiotics. May also be sexually transmitted.	Heavy, creamy, gray-white discharge that has a foul, fishy odor.	See a physician. Treatment is usually prescription drug Flagyl (metronidazole) in pill form.
Candidiasis (yeast infection)	Imbalance of natural vaginal bacteria due to diabetes, tight clothing, prolonged use of antibiotics such as tetracycline or birth control pills. Rarely sexually transmitted.	Thick, odorless, white discharge with the consistency of cottage cheese. Itching of the vulva and vagina and white patches of fungus over reddish, raw areas. Painful urination.	See a physician for correct diagnosis rather than trying to self-diagnose. Treatment of choice is either Monistat or Lotrimin in cream or suppository form. These are now available over-the-counter, but a correct diagnosis from your physician is crucial.
Tricho-moniasis	Caused by a protozoan organism spread via shared washcloths, towels, wet bathing suits or toilet seats. It is often sexually transmitted.	A frothy greenish-yellow, foul-smelling discharge, vaginal itching, inflammation of the vulva. There may also be frequent, painful urination and, in some cases, severe lower abdominal pain.	See a physician. The treatment is usually Flagyl in pill form. There are also Flagyl suppositories. Both forms are available only by prescription. If you're sexually active, your partner also needs to be treated.

■ Wash your genital area daily during your regular shower or bath.

■ Change your underwear daily and wear cotton or cotton-crotch underpants.

■ Don't share towels, washcloths or swimsuits.

■ Wipe yourself from front to back after a bowel movement. That way, you will avoid bringing any bacteria from the feces or anal area to your vaginal opening.

■ Don't use vaginal deodorant sprays or douches. These aren't necessary if you keep yourself clean with daily washing, and in fact can irritate the delicate tissues of the vulva and vagina. Frequent douching—cleansing the vagina with a water and vinegar mixture or a commercial douche solution—can disturb the normal acidic balance of the vagina, making vaginal infections *more* likely to happen.

Remember that a healthy vagina, with its normal discharge, cleans itself.

Coping With A Special Problem

When you have symptoms that tell you something is wrong, don't just hope these will go away. Tell your parents and your doctor.

You might be in for some very reassuring news. Physical changes that you think may be symptoms could turn out to be just normal changes of puberty. But it's always a good idea to check these out so you know for sure that you're in good health.

If your symptoms *are* a sign that something is wrong, the sooner you bring it to your parents' and doctor's attention, the sooner something can be done about it. You don't have to worry all alone. Whatever your problem is—whether it is one of the problems of puberty mentioned here or something less common or more serious—help is available.

Even if the help involves surgery or other uncomfortable treatments, it's important to remember that these treatments go on for a relatively short time—and, in many instances, bring you benefits for the rest of your life!

When you know there's help and hope, it can be a lot easier to cope with your problem—and then get on with the rest of your life!

10

How to Talk with Your Doctor (or School Nurse)

I hate going to the doctor! He has little kids running all over his waiting room. I feel like a baby going there. I have lots of questions I need to ask him, but I'm too scared to just come out and ask. He never asks me if I have any questions. Mostly, he just talks to my mom like I wasn't even there. How can I ask my doctor anything? ✳ BRIAN P.

What if I get my first period at school and have to go to the school nurse? I mean, what will I say? How do you act? What does she do? I'd be so embarrassed! I keep hoping and praying I get my first period at home, but what if I DO get it at school? ✳ SHERI G.

Talking to your doctor (or bringing up a concern or question to your school nurse) isn't always easy when you begin to grow up. When you were little, a parent probably did most of the talking and asking for you in the doctor's office. Now there may be some things you'd like to ask the doctor yourself—with or without a parent present. But, because all your physical changes are so new for you, you might feel self-conscious and embarrassed about asking your doctor anything. Or maybe you're afraid of bothering your doctor with a question he or she might consider silly.

If you find it difficult to talk to your doctor (or school nurse), here's some help. These are some of the most common problems young people have in talking to medical professionals—along with some ideas for asking what you need to know.

I'm So Embarrassed!

I want to ask my doctor if my breasts are growing O.K., but I'm embarrassed to ask him and embarrassed for him to see my breasts. What can I do? ✳ HILARY H.

If you've ever felt like Hilary does—you're far from alone! Asking your doctor about your body or having him or her do a physical exam isn't always easy when you're so aware of—and maybe a little self-conscious about—your changing body.

It may help to know that your doctor sees your body in a different way than you do. Although your doctor may care very much about your feelings and you as a person, he or she is looking at your body in a very scientific way to make sure that all is well. Also your doctor has seen hundreds, maybe thousands, of young people just like you. So there is probably very little that your doctor hasn't seen or heard.

If you're uncomfortable because you have a doctor of the opposite sex, say so. If the doctor knows you're feeling uneasy, he or she will usually take extra care to reassure you. If you truly can't deal with having a physician of the opposite sex, talk with your parents and see if it would be possible to change to a same-sex doctor. Opposite sex doctors *can* be just as sensitive to your problems as many same-sex doctors, but what matters most is your own comfort. If, despite everything your doctor does to help make an examination as easy as possible for you, you're still upset, it might make sense to try a same-sex doctor.

Most doctors, aware that you're especially concerned with privacy right now, will make an effort not to embarrass you during an examination. Usually, he or she will uncover only one area of your body at a time during a complete exam. And if you're especially shy about any particular area of your body, let the doctor know, so he or she can take extra care not to upset you.

For example, Jillian, who's 9, went to her doctor with a bad chest cold recently. When the nurse asked her to remove her blouse so the doctor could listen to her chest, Jillian said: "Could I have a drape or just leave my blouse open? I'm starting to get breasts and I feel sort of self-conscious." When the nurse and doctor realized how she felt, they were careful to expose as little of her breasts as possible. And her doctor asked her how she felt about beginning to grow up and if she had any questions she wanted to ask.

Asking a question that you're embarrassed to ask can be approached in the same way. Be honest about your feelings of embarrassment *and* your need for an answer: "Doctor, I feel embarrassed to ask this, but I really need to know—" Your doctor is likely to take it from there, helping you ask and then giving you the best answer he or she can.

Keep in mind that there are *no* dumb questions! In fact, it's smart to ask questions. A doctor likes to hear questions from you because it helps him or her help you!

If you find yourself in a situation you consider embarrassing—if, for example, you start your first menstrual period at school and go to the school nurse's office for a sanitary pad—the same is true. You really have to say very little because your school nurse has heard this many times before. She knows you may feel a little shy and, if she's like most, she'll try very hard to help you feel comfortable.

When Courtney, who is 11 and in the sixth grade, started her period at school recently, she went to the nurse's office and said "Miss Gage, I think I just started my first period." She was going to ask Miss Gage for a pad, but the nurse brought the supplies out, explained to Courtney how to remove the paper covering the adhesive strip and let her use the office bathroom privately to put on the first pad. That was all there was to it.

Of course, you may not end up seeing the school nurse if your school has sanitary napkin and tampon vending machines in the restroom or if you carry a mini-pad in your purse just in case you get your first period at school.

But do remember that whatever you need to ask your school nurse, she—like your doctor—has probably heard it before. You're not likely to shock her. She is there to help you the best way she can. And she knows that an important way medical professionals can aid young adolescents is to answer their questions and help them feel comfortable asking about—and living in—their changing bodies.

The Doctor Treats Me Like A Little Kid

I've been going to the same doctor since I was a baby and she still thinks I AM a baby! I can't stand it in her waiting room with little lambs and piggies all over the walls and screaming babies. Then, to top it all off, she keeps calling me Jackie when I really want to be called Jack because I'm almost 12. What can I do about this? ✳ JACK L.

You may be changing so fast that your doctor—and your parents— have trouble keeping up with how grown-up you really are!

If you're feeling babied at the doctor's office and you don't like it, here are some things you might do:

■ **Tell your doctor your preferences in a polite way.** The next time your doctor calls you by a childish nickname you hate, just say in a polite way, "Now that I'm almost grown-up, I'd rather be called—" or "Could you change my chart to read—" Your doctor won't know, unless you say so, what you really want to be called. Being assertive, in a respectful way, about your preferences is part of being grown-up.

■ **Participate in discussions with your doctor.** Little kids sit there passively and let their parents do all the talking. You can show that you're not a little kid anymore by volunteering information about symptoms or concerns when the doctor asks instead of just sitting there while your mom answers for you. If your doctor asks you a question, answer directly. And, if there is something he says that you don't understand, say so and ask him to explain. Speaking up on your own can help you get the information you need and can help others see that you're not a little kid. It tells your doctor and your parents that you're more mature now and want to be involved in your own health care.

■ **If the waiting room is like a nursery, ask about special hours.** If you hate sharing the waiting room with babies and small children, ask your doctor if he has special hours for adolescents or if he would consider such scheduling. Many doctors do.

■ **If your doctor doesn't seem to like treating teenagers, try another doctor.** Some doctors are more comfortable with little kids, and some enjoy young adults the most. You might ask your parents about going to one with a specialty in adolescent medicine. These doctors treat only mature preteens and teenagers and are often especially interested in helping you feel good about your changing body.

The Doctor Is So Busy!

My problem with my doctor is that whenever I get the nerve to ask him what I need to ask, he's walking out the door. Or else I forget until I'm halfway home. How can I ask him anything when he's so busy? I feel funny about bothering him, but there's some stuff I really need to know! ✳ MELISSA M.

Many young people have this frustrating problem. If this has happened to you, here's what you can do: Write out a list of your questions before going to the doctor. This will help you remember what to ask. If you're embarrassed, *read* the questions to your doctor.

A good way to make sure that your doctor has time to answer your questions: Make an appointment just to talk and ask what you need to know; or tell your doctor at the beginning of the appointment that there are some questions you would like to ask. You might even show him or her the list. That might help you get started.

Some teens and preteens expect their doctors to be mind readers, able to guess when they have something they want to discuss. Sometimes that happens, but, quite often, unless you come out and ask, your doctor won't realize what your special concerns are. And you'll feel disappointed and frustrated. So don't go to the doctor complaining about headaches if your real concern is about an uncomfortable vaginal discharge.

Tell your doctor what you need to know. Both of you will be happier. You will get the answers you need, and he or she will have the satisfaction of helping you.

I Want To Talk To The Doctor Alone

This is a tough problem, at least for me. I am a boy who's 12 and I live with my mom. I almost never see my dad anymore. (My parents were divorced when I was 2.) Well, when I go to the doctor, which isn't often, I have some things I want to ask him. But some of it is embarrassing to talk about in front of my mom, who's always there. It's not like I'm doing anything wrong. But I wanted to ask the doctor about whether I'm maturing O.K. (I'm scared about my penis being small) and about wet dreams I've heard about but which haven't happened to me yet. How can I ask to talk to my doctor alone without hurting my mom's feelings? ✻ SHAWN F.

If you want some time alone with your doctor, try talking about this need with your parent first. That way, your request for a private consultation will not come as a surprise or seem like a rejection.

For example, Shawn might tell his mother that, now that he's growing up, he has some questions about his physical changes that he feels most comfortable discussing with another man. His mother, who may be able to remember when she was growing up and felt shy about her father knowing everything about her changes, will probably be able to understand right away. If she doesn't, Shawn might reassure her that he still feels close to her and loves her a lot, but just doesn't feel comfortable right now talking with or in front of her about all his physical changes.

When you go to the doctor, your parent might stay in the waiting room or leave you alone for a few minutes at the end of the appointment. You might ask the doctor, at the beginning of your visit, if you can have some time alone. That way, the doctor may help remind you and your parent about this request if your parent seems to forget and you're reluctant to make a big deal out of it.

While it's wonderful if you can share most, if not all, of your feelings, questions and experiences with your parents, there may be times when you need another opinion or feel that you can't talk about your physical development with someone who is very close to you. Some people need more privacy than others, but it's O.K. to keep some questions between yourself and your doctor.

Other young people feel just the opposite: They *want* a parent with them in the doctor's office. That's fine, too. What's most important is what makes you feel comfortable and able to learn about your body and your health.

Some young people, particularly those who live in cities and have working parents, may go to the doctor alone for routine camp or sports physicals. If you visit your doctor for an exam on your own, be sure to remember to bring a permission note from your parents for any blood test or immunization you might need. There are times when a doctor can't sign your physical report for sports participation or camp without having given you a certain immunization. And shots can't be given unless you have written permission from your parents. So remembering that note can save you a lot of time and frustration!

The Doctor Asks Me Too Many Questions!

I have a problem. I clam up in the doctor's office, even though I have questions I'd like to ask. One of the problems is I'm sort of shy. The other problem is that the doctor asks too many questions. It makes me mad. Why does she ask so many questions? ❋ JANELLE E.

Some of the questions a doctor asks you may seem dumb. But your honest answers can help your physician get an accurate picture of your health and find ways to help you avoid major problems and risks.

A doctor is likely to ask you about:

■ **Your family health history.** He or she is trying to find out whether certain medical conditions known to run in families are present in *your* family. That's why he or she may ask whether anyone in your family has had diabetes, asthma, high blood pressure, kidney disease, heart disease or allergies.

■ **Your immunization records.** Your doctor wants to make sure you're up-to-date on all the important immunization shots. It's easy to dismiss them as just a nuisance. But some of these immunizations are really important to your health. Your parents or grandparents may be able to tell you what it was like not that long ago when there was no vaccine protection against polio—and thousands of young people lost their lives or were crippled for life. Or how devastating common diseases such as measles were for some people. These diseases are still around, so it's very important to protect yourself against them.

Immunizations Alert!
Missing Anything?

The U.S. Centers for Disease Control estimate that 35 million U.S. adolescents could be missing at least one of the recommended vaccinations necessary to safeguard health through the teen and young adult years.

Which immunizations should you have and when?

By age 12:   Three doses of hepatitis B vaccine

Second dose of measles-mumps-rubella (MMR) vaccine

Varicella (chickenpox) vaccine

By age 16:   All of the above plus tetanus and diphtheria toxoid (td)

If You're Not Protected . . .

You're in danger of getting hepatitis B, which is:

■ A serious infection of the liver that can lead to chronic disease, cancer and death.

■ 100 times more contagious than the virus that causes AIDS.

■ Caught by blood contact that includes infection acquired through contact sports; sharing an infected person's earrings, toothbrush or razor; getting a tattoo or ear or body piercing with nonsterile equipment; contact with a surface contaminated by infected blood or body fluids (Hepatitis B can remain infectious on some surfaces for as long as a week!); or sexual contact.

■ Usually acquired during the teen or early adult years. 17 percent of new hepatitis B infections occur in those 10 to 19 years of age. Those infected as teens have a 15 percent change of dying from liver disease.

Would You Believe . . .

From 50 to 70 percent of all adolescents have not yet been protected against hepatitis B!!!

Are You One Of Them???

Talk To Your Doctor Today!!

■ **Major diseases and common complaints.** To get a thorough health history, your doctor needs to know if you've had measles, mumps, chicken pox, German measles (rubella), allergies, pneumonia, bronchitis, tonsillitis and whether you have chronic conditions such as diabetes or epilepsy. He or she may also ask you whether and how often you tend to have: colds, a sore throat, headaches, dizziness, ear infections, constipation, diarrhea, excessive thirst, unexplained weight loss or gain, difficulty in concentrating or any other problems that concern you.

Your doctor will also want to know if—and why—you've ever been hospitalized, what prescription drugs you are currently taking and if you're sensitive to any particular drug (e.g., penicillin).

■ **Your personal habits.** When a doctor asks you if you eat breakfast or if you smoke, drink or take drugs, he or she isn't trying to be nosy—or insult you. Good eating habits are important to your health. And potentially harmful habits such as smoking, drinking and drug use can also affect your health a lot. Sadly, such habits are not unknown among preteens and that's why your doctor may ask you about it.

■ **Your physical development.** If you have a new doctor, he may ask you when you began to develop physically. If you've been to this doctor regularly, he may simply ask how things are going for you.

This is all just a way to make sure that your growth and development are progressing and that you're not having any unusual problems. For example, if you're a girl and have already started to menstruate, the doctor will probably ask when you had your last period, if your periods are regular, if you have cramps, premenstrual symptoms and whether the flow is light, medium or heavy. Even though it may seem that the doctor is being nosy, he or she isn't trying to discover all the secrets of your life, just facts that relate to the general state of your health.

What if *you* have questions you want to ask, but these get lost in the flurry of the doctor's questions?

There are several things you can do. First, after you have answered the doctor's questions, say: "May I ask you something now? There's something I need to know." Or, when the doctor is questioning you and gets to an area where you have a special concern, you might bring it up then. For example, if he asks you about your menstrual periods, now could be a good time to bring up any questions or concerns you have about that.

Asking questions helps your doctor learn more about you and give you better medical care. When you ask questions, you're also learning. Most doctors *prefer* that you ask questions. Those who ask questions are seen as intelligent and involved, not silly or dumb or troublesome.

To best understand your body and your medical care, it's important to get into the habit of asking questions not only about your growth, development and general health but also about any medical treatments, medicines or tests you're getting.

If you don't understand a doctor's directions, ask questions until you do understand. Ask him why certain tests or medications are being given. Will the tests hurt? Do the medications have side effects? How can you help to increase the effectiveness of the treatment? How long should you take medications?

The better you understand what's going on with your body and with your health care, the better you and your doctor will communicate. Once you understand each other, you'll realize that you're both part of a team—to help you enjoy a lifetime of good health!

11

How to Talk with Your Parents

I'm 9 years old and have lots of questions about growing up. I'd like to talk with my mom, except I don't know how to bring it all up. She never says anything. How can I just ask her? ✳ JENNIFER T.

I tried to talk with my dad last night about developing and stuff. We didn't get anywhere. He got all nervous and started telling me about birds, bees and babies. I've known about that for ages. What I wanted to know was about what's happening with my body right now and what to expect. I figured he'd been through it. But you'd never know it. How can I ask him about things that are important to me? ✳ MIKE L.

What do you do if you try to ask your parents questions about growing up, only they're always too busy to tell you anything? ✳ NICOLE A.

These letters reveal some of the most common problems preteens and their parents have in communicating about growing and changing. These can be difficult times for preteens *and* for their parents.

Watching a child growing so rapidly can make parents happy and sad at the same time. They're happy to see you growing up, but sad to see you growing away. Sometimes they're not sure how to treat you— or what you really need to know.

"I'm fascinated and also a little unsure of myself when I look at my 10-year-old daughter," one father told us recently. "I'm not quite sure whether she's a large child or a small woman . . . or somewhere in between. It's not easy to know how to be with her or know what she needs. Sometimes she's very adult. At other times, she's a little girl again."

As you grow through this in-between time, talking about your physical changes may not always be easy for you or your parents. Yet there are probably a lot of questions you'd like to ask.

How can you start asking your parents what you need to know?

Here are the most common problems preteens face in talking with their parents—and some ideas for starting to share questions, thoughts and feelings in a new way.

I'm Too Embarrassed To Ask . . . They're Too Embarrassed To Tell Me Anything!

If you're too embarrassed to ask your parents anything, remember—as hard as it may be to imagine—that your parents once went through the very same changes you're experiencing now. So they know how it is.

It may surprise them to know that you're changing so fast, but they can help you in a special way. They can give you a lot more than simply factual information. Because they know you so well and care about you so much, they can give you information and guidance that's just right for you.

Of course, sometimes being close and caring so much can make it difficult to start talking. As many young people have told us, at times it's easier to write a letter asking intimate questions to a stranger than it is to ask a loved one. But once you get over your initial embarrassment, you and your parents will have a lot to share!

If you're too embarrassed to bring up a topic, tell your parents about someone you know or something you've read as a way of easing into your question.

For example, if Jennifer knows a classmate, friend or a friend's older sister who recently started menstruating, she could say to her mother: "Mom, a girl named Tracey, who's in my class, got her period already. It makes me think about growing up and I wonder when I'll start menstruating. I really want to ask you some questions now . . ."

Another way to get communication going between you and your parent is to bring the parent a book and ask your questions based on that. For example, "I'm confused about what I've read here. What do *you* think?" Or "It says in this book that children's growth and development can be a lot like that of their parents. Do you remember when you started growing up? How old were you? What can I expect to happen to me in a year or so?"

Books can also help if your parent is too embarrassed to talk about development, growth and sexuality. You might, for example, ask for his or her help in finding the right books or pamphlets that will teach you what you want to know. That way, you can share the search for good information and still feel close. Reading books together may help you and your parent begin talking eventually. Your parent may be able to explain things you don't understand in a book or may have some opinions about what is written. This can be the beginning of a new kind of sharing.

My Parents Are Too Busy

This is a common complaint in these days when every family member has a busy schedule and most parents work outside the home.

The best way to get around frantic schedules: Ask your parents for time before you start asking questions!

You might say something like "Do you have time to talk now?" Tell them that there are some questions you need to ask. Let them know that this is important to you. If now is a bad time, ask them when they might have time to talk. Make an appointment if necessary. But do let your parents know that you need them.

Another way to catch up with busy parents is to join them in a work project or activity and talk with them then. You might be amazed at some of the good talks you can have with a parent while helping with yard work or taking a walk.

An 11-year-old named Kirsten tells us that she has learned a lot in conversations with her mother during after-dinner walks. "It works out well because she can't see me blushing when I ask her something embarrassing so I don't feel quite so embarrassed—if that makes any sense," she says. "We've been getting lots of exercise and having really good talks. My mom's a lawyer and when she first comes home, she's really tired and tense. But she relaxes as we walk and that makes it easier for her to listen to me and to help me."

With a little planning and a lot of caring, you and your parents can make time for each other in your own special ways.

My Parents Never Tell Me What I Need To Know!

If they're talking birds and bees and you want to know something more specific, ask a specific question!

Chances are, your parents are too close to you to realize how quickly you're growing up. They may not be able to anticipate or bring up what you need to know. Also, they aren't mind readers. If you ask vague questions, they may simply have to guess what it is you *really* want to know.

If, for example, you tell your mom or dad that you need more information about growing up, your parent may react in one of several ways. If you're especially lucky, he or she might ask you what you particularly need to know. Or your parent might launch into a discussion of what he or she *thinks* you want to know.

If your mom or dad has guessed right, great! If not, thank him or her for that information and then ask as clearly as you can what you really want to know.

These are a few specific questions some preteens we know asked their parents recently:

■ "Is it normal for your breasts to hurt a little when they're first growing?"

■ "When should I start using a deodorant? Do you think I'm old enough now?"

■ "Is it unusual to start liking girls before you're a teenager?"

■ "How will I know if my first menstrual period will be coming soon?"

When a parent hears a question as specific as these, it's easier for him or her to give you the answer you need.

A lot of these questions, of course, are answered in this book. But talking with your parents can be especially helpful because they know you so well.

Some preteens—and parents, too—put off trying to talk about subjects they think are embarrassing until they feel comfortable talking about it. The problem is, if you wait until you feel totally comfortable to start talking about growth, development and sexuality with each other, you may wait forever! And you could miss a lot of good information and a chance to share important thoughts and feelings with each other.

So even though you're feeling embarrassed or unsure, reach out to each other—even if it's to share your feelings of embarrassment! If you can say "I'm kind of embarrassed to talk about this . . ." and your parent can say "Me, too . . . but let's give it a try!" you may both end up relaxing a little and feeling more comfortable right away!

It's important to help each other along. Your parents might help by asking you if you want to talk or if you have any more questions. You can help by letting your parents know that you appreciate their efforts—even if they're really nervous talking about such things. Helping each other in this way may make your next talk and those to follow much easier.

There are some families who find the subject of growing up and sexuality simply impossible to discuss. If that's the case in your home, there are other places you can get important information: books, magazines, health education classes, talking with the school nurse or your doctor or other relatives and adult friends.

But if it's at all possible, talking with your parents can be well worth any special effort it takes. Your parents care for you more than anyone else. They want the very best for you now and in the future. And now is the best possible time to start reaching out to each other with love and understanding!

12

Growing Toward New Discoveries

I'm getting interested in boys. But lots of boys in my class are SO gross! I mean, they think it's really funny to just stand around making disgusting noises all the time! Some of them are just awful when they get together, but O.K. if you're just talking to one of them. Why is that? I'd really like to have a special boyfriend, but they all act embarrassing! ✳ ELISA P.

I don't understand girls at all. They get mad if you tease them about anything. And they're super-paranoid about their bodies. Like you can't say anything or they get all upset. I'd like to have a girlfriend. But how can I talk to her without getting her mad or upset? ✳ JARED R.

During these growing years, you'll start noticing the opposite sex more and more.

First, you'll notice the differences.

Maybe the girls are taller and heavier than a lot of the guys and seem more mature. And because they are very conscious of their new physical changes, they are very sensitive if teased about their bodies.

Boys, who often begin developing a bit later than girls, may not yet feel such self-consciousness. They want to be noticed, but look for attention in ways that *they* (and their male friends) think are appropriate—making weird or rude noises or teasing.

Boys and girls grow and change in different ways. Your bodies look different in shape and size. But are you *really* that different?

Boys and girls, men and women—all are more alike than different. We're all people who:

■ sometimes worry and wonder about being normal

■ have tender feelings that can be hurt

■ find body changes and new sexual feelings confusing, fascinating and important

■ want to be liked by others

■ think that having friends is *very* important

■ want to have someone special to love and share a variety of feelings and experiences with

So even though our bodies differ in some ways, many of our feelings are very much the same! That's why, especially during this time in between childhood and young adulthood, it's important to be as caring and kind as you can.

Be kind to yourself. That's *very* important. Don't criticize yourself constantly if your body isn't exactly perfect. Your body is wonderful in its own unique way. It can bring you a lot of pleasure if you treat it well and learn to like and accept it. Don't consider yourself a failure if you're not immediately popular with girls or boys. It takes time to get comfortable with each other. It takes time to know yourself well enough to discover what kind of special person you'd like to grow to love one day.

Be kind to others, too. Even those who act gross or seem confident and cool have their own fears, questions and insecurities about growing up.

Sometimes girls think that boys don't have feelings because they're not as likely to show hurt or pain as girls might be. But boys *do* get hurt by put-downs and rejections. And girls, who may seem so different, are really a lot like boys. They worry about physical changes and wonder what's going on. They're anxious and scared and excited, just as boys are at times about growing up.

Differences between males and females are especially noticeable now as you begin to see the opposite sex in a new way. But look at each other a little closer—beyond those differences in your height or weight or shape or level of maturity. You'll see people who are mostly just like you: people who can be wonderful friends.

As you begin to discover boys and girls as people, you'll touch each other's lives in a special new way—with friendship and with love!

Cool Stuff for Browsing

TEENS GROWTH

www.teensgrowth.com

This is a great website that gives you all kinds of information you want and need to make sure that your teen years are healthy, fun and safe. Special note for people who hate math and charts: You can calculate your body mass index as well as your probable adult height via the special online calculator.

KIDS HEALTH

www.kidshealth.org

An excellent source of information for every physical and emotional health question you could have in either English or Spanish. It includes very complete and understandable answers to some of the questions most asked by pre-teens and teens such as "What's the right weight for my height?" and "How can I lose weight safely?"

ADOLESCENT HEALTH INFORMATION FROM BOSTON CHILDREN'S HOSPITAL AND HARVARD UNIVERSITY

www.youngwomenshealth.org/healthinfo.html

Bookmark this site today—whether you're male or female! Although there *is* a lot of info here on matters of most interest to girls—like menstruation and gynecological health—there is also a lot of great information about topics of interest to preteens and teens of both sexes, including good nutrition (including creative ideas for nutritious backpack snacks), eating disorders, dealing with a parental divorce, depression, friendship, body piercing, vegetarianism, sports, scoliosis and an array of other teen topics. This site even offers a downloadable order form if you're interested in buying its new cookbook *Quick and Easy Recipes for Teens*.

PUBERTY 101
www.puberty101.com
This comprehensive teen mental and physical health site answers your questions no matter how weird you think they are. It's a good place to check out what other teens and preteens are asking—and to get good information from an adolescent counselor. There are also online illustrations that help you to understand your body and the changes of puberty.

ADOLESCENCE DIRECTORY ONLINE
www.education.indiana.edu/cas/adol/adol.html
Talk about a one-stop comprehensive site! This website is an electronic treasure chest for teens that includes 'zines, a directory to fun sites and honest, reliable help with a variety of questions and problems about your health and your life. But that's not all! You can actually get help with your math homework (no matter what grade you're in or level of difficulty your math class is) through this site's Dr. Math, and you can do all kinds of research on colleges, getting frank comments from current students there, at the College Edge.

SOCIETY FOR ADOLESCENT MEDICINE
www.adolescenthealth.org
While it's mostly for medical professionals who specialize in adolescent health, this site also has a special feature for teens called "Tips for Teens" that gives excellent information on topics such as anger management, substance abuse, depression and suicide, getting good health care and stress management. It also offers links to sites covering a wide variety of teen health and other topics of interest to teens.

TEENS LIFE AND HEALTH DIGEST
www.aizan.net/families/teens.htm
This site includes hotlines and information about a variety of health and lifestyle-related issues including parent-teen relationships, careers and self-help quizzes.

FAMILY DOCTOR
www.familydoctor.org/teens.html
Very helpful information here about making important decisions in your life and how to manage stress as well as a variety of other health challenges.

NEW MOON'ZINE
www.newmoon.org
This is a bimonthly online magazine for girls ages 8 to 14. Lots of good stuff!

JUNIOR MED
www.juniormed.com
This is an online health library with topics of interest to preteens and their parents.

KIDSOURCE
www.kidsource.com
This site offers information on everything from immunizations to safe use of motorized scooters.

AMERICAN MEDICAL ASSOCIATION
www.ama-assn.org/ama/pub/category/1947.html
The American Medical Association site offers great information on adolescent health *and* a handy "Physician Finder" search feature that allows you to search for a doctor by name or by specialty.

THE TEENAGE BODY BOOK (KATHY MCCOY, PH.D., AND CHARLES WIBBELSMAN, M.D.)
www.theteenagebodybook.com
Visit us at our new website for all kinds of additional information on your health and other problems, pleasures or challenges in your life. It's a chance for you to ask a question directly and get a personal answer!

Index

Page numbers in *italic* indicate illustrations; those in **bold** indicate charts or tables.